Minus One

Dorothy Hansen

Minus One

a year with breast cancer

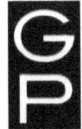

Acknowledgements

The author and publisher make grateful acknowledgement to the following for permission to use copyright material:

Elizabeth Bishop and Chatto & Windus for lines from 'One Art'; the late Shelton Lea and Black Pepper for 'i dream of the soft slide of light'; Ian McEwan and Jonathan Cape for the extract from *Saturday*; Les Murray and William Heinemann Australia for lines from 'The Broad Bean Sermon'; Mary Oliver and Beacon Press for 'Why I wake Early' and lines from 'Mindful'; and M.Scott Peck and Simon & Schuster for the extract from *In Search of Stones*.

Minus One: a year with breast cancer
ISBN 978 1 74027 469 2
Copyright © text Dorothy Hansen 2007
Cover design: Bruce Edwards, detail from untitled painting by the late Jean Appleton, in the possession of the author

First published 2007
Reprinted 2017

GINNINDERRA PRESS
PO Box 3461 Port Adelaide 5015
www.ginninderrapress.com.au

When I go from hence, let this be my parting word,
that what I have seen is unsurpassable.

          Rabindranath Tagore, *Gitanjali*

1

November

On the way to the operating theatre I found that to my surprise I was remarkably calm. On reflection I remember with extraordinary clarity every detail of the cubicle where I waited before being wheeled into the bright lights of this strange, exotic world where I would go in whole but come out minus one – minus one breast.

There was almost an inevitability about this moment in time. For twenty-five years I had lived with the thought that one day I might not be so fortunate. On my twenty-fifth wedding anniversary I had waited anxiously with my husband outside a specialist's rooms. My GP had told me he thought my lump was likely to be cancerous. But it seemed so large and I was quite sure it hadn't been there two weeks before. To our utter delight it was aspirated by the surgeon and we celebrated our silver wedding with added pleasure. Ever since, I have had cysts aspirated at fairly regular intervals. Only in the last few years had they become less frequent but I had mammograms, sometimes ultrasounds and breast examinations. All to prevent what was now happening to me. I didn't go along with friends who spoke of life events as 'being meant to be'. How do we part easily from something that is part of who we are? It was thirty years since my womb had been removed. Suddenly. Just like this breast. Why did it all have to be done in a hurry?

I had rushed to the shops and bought a couple of attractive nighties to add to my rather unglamorous collection. That didn't really seem to matter now. I had missed the opportunity to lavish attention on my wardrobe. There had always been so much to do. So many books to complete. One of my sons, now an art gallery curator, was finishing off the details of his Litt.D. to be awarded by Melbourne University. He lived in Hobart but insisted that he come over 'to look after Dad'. He and his father were alike in many ways and I knew I didn't have to worry about them. I had packed some books, and bought myself a new toilet bag. Nothing seemed important, somehow. I just wanted to get it all over and done with.

And now I wafted off into some strange country to be woken up by a kind nursing sister. I seemed to be the only person left in the recovery unit and eventually I was taken to my room. My two men had been concerned about me, I was told later. Our son David had made a valiant attempt to amuse his father by endeavouring to translate into French a Tim Winton short story they had been reading. There was no pain for me, just a feeling of light-headedness probably caused by me pushing the pain relief button subconsciously. It was a relief to know that it was all over. They had taken my lymph nodes (thirteen, I was told by a sensitive male nurse some days later), and only one was cancerous. I didn't know how to tell my husband, my lover for so many years. He is four years older than me and I had always thought I would be there for him and now I was expecting him to deal with this. Each night as we said goodnight to each other on the telephone I found it hard to hang up. The connection between the two of us is something I never cease to marvel at. He is a poet, and had brought me a poem in a letter when he came in to see me. It seemed to say all the things he felt.

Storm
(for Dorothy)

Fear creeps into the cave
that we've dug to keep us
warm against the thrashing winds
and the rain that thunders.

It's dark here and we wait
We cling together and gusts
tug at us. And yet there is something
that comes unbidden and near,

Like an embrace that folds us both.
There is now with this dread,
and a then full of memory,
and what is to follow we want to know.

At night's end the trees are still,
the grass wet and green,
and light from the east stirs.
We let each other go and search

our faces and find a serene
and persisting hope that tells
of tearing rags of cloud
that let in the beckoning blue of sky.

    My surgeon came in every day, read my charts and checked my drainage bottle. Fortunately, the sight of blood has never upset me. The only problem was taking the bottle with its tube attached when I went to the shower each morning.

    Mornings have never been my best time. I had always worked best late in the day when everyone else was sensibly in bed. So I hadn't seen hundreds of dawns. Those I had seen I remembered. In Geneva once, badly jet-lagged, I had stood at our hotel room window and as the light came over the rooftops watched the men in a nearby bakery busy making the day's bread. In London when the children were young we had all got up early to go to the old Covent Garden market: I had wanted them to experience the noise and frantic activity that is part of all markets, but the children had come to buy the promised strawberries to take back home for breakfast. On the first morning after surgery I had wakened as the early light crept over the city. A flock of birds flew past etched against the soft pink, white and grey of the sky. So good it was to be alive, to hear the stirring of a busy world outside my quiet room. I breathed deeply of the morning air. A new day.

    David, the Hobart son, had brought me a collection of poems by the American poet Mary Oliver. I reached over to my bedside table, attracted to one entitled 'Why I wake early'.

Hello, sun in my face,
Hello, you who make the morning
and spread it over the fields
and into the faces of tulips
and the nodding morning glories,
and into the windows of, even, the
miserable and the crotchety-

best preacher that ever was,
dear star that just happens
to be where you are in the universe
to keep us from ever-darkness,
to ease us with warm touching,
to hold us in the great hands of light-
good-morning, good morning, good morning.

Watch now, how I start the day
in happiness, in kindness.

    It is the little things in life that warm us in the dark days and nights. When I arrived back in my room from surgery, there was a beautiful arrangement of yellow roses waiting there. They had come from friends we had met while holidaying in France. The blooms glowed in the morning light.

    Each morning the South American cleaning lady came in with her bright smile, admired and seemed very knowledgeable about each flower arrangement. She had become the one person I could depend upon seeing each morning. Nurses changed with great regularity. I rarely saw them more than once. But the cleaning lady did more for the well-being of patients than she would ever know.

    Visitors always seemed to come in groups and I found myself introducing them to each other and trying to be a hostess in a room with few chairs. The days didn't seem too long. There was always something happening and now I was able to walk around the corridors with my bottle. It seemed to connect me, if only ever so slightly, to a larger world than my hospital room.

    I looked at the scar as the blood ran along the tube and drained into the collecting jar. I was thankful it was the left breast they had removed. I can do so much more with my right hand and have always slept on my right side. I thought about scars. After a recent severe storm, one of the branches had sheared off one of our giant gum trees in the back garden. It too had bled where the great branch left the main trunk.

I have met people who seem to have few life scars, who have never been wounded or shaken in body, mind or spirit. I find that often they seemed to understand little about life at depth, have rarely questioned the meaning of life, seem safe in their own protected world. People speak of 'the wounded healer'. Perhaps they are right and we can only heal from our own place of vulnerability and pain.

Wandering around Florence some years ago, I had looked long and hard at the sculpture by Verrochio outside the church of Orsanmichele. St Thomas is standing there with his hand stretched out but unable, it seems, to touch the place of the scar. Christ's hand is raised as if to say, 'It's all right, Thomas.' My scar needed to be felt even with the dark stitches still showing. The first time I washed it under the shower I physically winced. Not from pain but from the sight of it.

I have been thoroughly spoilt. One son and his partner have given me the softest spun wool wrap to put around my shoulders, my granddaughter bought me a pretty pair of pyjamas covered with red lilies and my country son and his fiancée travelled eight and a half hours by car to visit me.

I know that I am still euphoric with the happiness of post-surgery days, but I am so thankful to be alive. I was told that my drainage tube would come out the day before I went home. I hadn't been looking forward to the experience but a wise nursing sister came in an hour before it was due to be removed and, before I could become tense thinking about it, it was out in a few seconds and I felt free at last. Tomorrow I would be going home to begin life with a different future. A future minus one.

My three children had grown up with the bathroom door always open unless they chose to close it. It had always amused me the way in which as they grew older they would come in and stand in the doorway talking to me in the bath about all manner of things. And so it was now. Both the boys said, 'Give us a look at your scar, Mum.' There was a naturalness about it. With my hysterectomy almost thirty years ago, there had been nothing to see, and in any case we were so involved in so many things that I had scarcely been aware of my discomfort. Now the boys were older. They wanted to see my violation. I was proud of their sensitivity and their ease about my lopsidedness.

It would be a couple of months before I could get my prosthesis but the hospital had given me a soft 'breast' to place in my ordinary bras until then. To the outsider there was nothing to see. I was surprised that people weren't conscious of the fact that when they knew of my surgery their eyes immediately went to my breasts. The scar line seemed to come just where my bras sat. It would all have been so much easier to deal with had the scar not extended under my arm. The stitches still had to dissolve and there was a numbness remaining but, provided that I didn't sleep on my left side, I was able to sleep well.

The chemotherapy tablets I take after dinner each evening produce in me a warm flush three hours almost to the minute after they are taken. What an extraordinary thing the human body is. What a marvel of engineering. That each night my body would respond in this way. It lasted for only a short time, but that it should happen with such unerring timing was in itself a small miracle.

I think each morning as I stand in the bathroom looking down at the cavern where my breast once was that it is the daily reminder that is the problem. This gaping hole has been the memory place of babies and my lover's hands. There is no way to escape what for me was now so aesthetically displeasing. I have been asked if I want a breast reconstruction but there are for me more important things I want to be getting on with. Time for Ian, the children, grandchildren, friends. I can understand the young women who opt for a reconstruction. Had I been in my thirties or forties, I would probably have gone ahead with it but not at this time of my life.

There are times in the early recovery period when I feel that the therapy has scrambled my brain. I have been looking at a documentary on the life of Alfred Kinsey and was reminded of his research on the gall wasp. So patiently over a period of time he had collected thousands of samples of this creature. I think that they are quite stunning to look at, all those tiny creatures. But not one of them was exactly like another. So with chemotherapy responses. They were going to be slightly different for everyone.

As the weeks go by, I am sure I am returning to something like my former self. There are days when quite involuntarily my eyes fill with tears in response to my inner grief and loss, but that is probably true of many women in my situation. It isn't the surgery that is the problem, it is the aftermath. I resist going to a group at this stage. I'm not ready to embrace any one else's pain or reveal mine. That will probably come later.

I do my exercises religiously each day. The one thing I had asked the surgeon was that he should not do anything to prevent me from playing the piano. All my life I have turned to it when I wanted to escape the world and it is the source of so much energy for me. As a small girl I had pleaded with my parents to learn the piano and so at seven years of age I had lessons and have been playing ever since. I had been told I was a good accompanist while I was still at school. I accompanied the school choir for an ABC broadcast, had even thought that I could perhaps make a living from it, but instead I had begun my working life as a research librarian and music took second place. But I was never without it. It would always be a strong part of who I am.

Ian and I had been given a grand piano in 1960 while we were living in London. We were returning home and by sea and this enabled us to bring it home. There was a strike at the wharf in England and the crates waited there in the summer heat for several weeks. The day it was ready for delivery in Melbourne I just had to leave the house until it was unpacked. I couldn't bear the thought of it being damaged in any way. The beautiful rosewood case still gleamed as it had in 1852 when it was crafted and after tuning it played Bach and Beethoven with an almost original sound, I thought. Playing the piano seems to be good for my arm and certainly I have no ill effects from it. I can lose myself in music and forget about everything else.

All the booklets said to be careful of scratches to the arm, insect bites and so on and I didn't give it much thought until I went out to pick a bunch of roses from the garden and was aware of the sharp prickles on the bushes. I took great care with them as I placed them in the basket. I certainly didn't want the dreaded lymphodoema that the booklets spoke of in such detail.

I am not a logical housewife. Each morning I do the flowers before anything else. If the house has fresh flowers in it it seems to come alive and there is always something to pick and some foliage to add to whatever flowers are blooming.

I notice in these early weeks that if I am in a crowd I instinctively move my left arm away from where it might be knocked by a passer-by. It isn't an intentional act, more like the body protecting itself. I try to listen to my body. If I feel tired I will rest for a bit. I am not yet able to do heavy lifting or vacuuming and Ian watches me like a hawk to make sure I don't take any risks.

Because the weather is getting warmer I felt sure the sunshine would speed up the healing process and being able to walk around the block in the cool evenings make me conscious of all the changes going on in my nearby physical landscape. Houses are continually being added to, pulled down, painted and renovated. I have never understood people who wanted nips and tucks. Perhaps I was just a coward. Why have surgery when you didn't have to?

My physical map has changed. The contours have changed. There is now a deep gully and a slight hill where once there had been the generous curves of a breast. I had been rather flat-chested until well after my three children were born. I suppose I should have paid more attention to my physical body, but life was always so rich, so full. Now I had to make time for it.

2

January

I had been told in the hospital that after two months I should get my prosthesis. What I had been given in hospital was only a temporary affair, light, and filled with soft nylon-looking stuffing encased in a cotton 'breast'.

The government is generous in its subsidy. It was just that yet again there was someone looking at my one remaining breast and trying to find the right match for it with the prosthesis. The shopgirl was charming and did everything she could to put me at ease. In they came – various sizes and all looking like chicken fillets. It was still summer and the cubicle was hot, or was I hot and bothered? It all seemed to be taking such a long time to find the right one and meanwhile I could hear people talking in other cubicles. Talking about bras for nursing mothers and 'normal' bras. We walk around and observe the young flaunting their pretty breasts, see babies tugging at their mothers' breasts when they want a feed, and rightly don't imagine for one moment that there are people wearing a false breast that, although it is similar in weight to the other breast, feels like a sack of apples or potatoes and doesn't seem to give as you walk.

Ian had been the one I had worried about. How would he react to the sight of me naked? After I came home from hospital I had quickly undressed and was in bed before he came into the room. He was so positive about everything. So anxious to make me feel that loving was accepting and that so long as I was there beside him nothing else mattered. But for his sake I longed to be as I had been before surgery. Just for fun I had sometimes done my Marilyn Monroe act as

I undressed and we had laughed together about my now fuller breasts. I can't do any of that any more.

Putting on my new bras each morning is yet another reminder of how it is going to be from now on. I know that in time it will just become a matter of course. Ian had been diagnosed with coeliac disease twelve months earlier. This meant no wheat, rye, oats or barley. For the first few weeks we read every label, checked every purchase in the supermarket. But now we could shop with our usual speed knowing what could be eaten and what not. I suppose it will be the same thing with my prosthesis. All a matter of time.

At the moment I feel dried up inside. It is as if my life's juices aren't flowing. I remembered walking along the banks of the Lachlan with my son on our last visit before my operation to the property he managed. At this particular bend, the river had nothing left in it but squelching mud. It no longer acted as a fence for the sheep and a large ewe had managed to get down the bank and was struggling with the weight of its fleece to even stand up. The relentless heat beat down on us and my son scrambled down to set the ewe free. There was the odd shower of rain and when it came no one bothered to shelter from it. The clouds would gather and then disperse and the waiting farmers continued to hand feed.

I feel as if I am waiting for rain. I can't explain my lack of buoyancy. It is as if I am in drought, waiting for the refreshing rains to come and restore my equilibrium. I feel as out of balance as the ewe and who is going to come and lift me out of the mud? I had been on a low dose of hormone replacement therapy ever since my hysterectomy and the debate had raged in medical circles about the advisability of taking it for long periods of time. Now I am off it I wonder whether all my drive and energy was related to my hormones and whether it is simply the body adjusting.

I am to see my surgeon every three months and on the advice of a young GP friend, I make an appointment with an oncologist. I want to know whether I am on the best medication and I have heard good reports of the comparatively new drug, Arimidex. The oncologist is sensitive and didn't rush through my pathology reports. He did his calculations and told me what percentage in my age group and with a cancerous lymph node were still alive in five years and in ten years. I needed to know. I was determined to be positive and be one of the survivors.

To change my medication I am required to have a bone density test because the new drug had affected bones in some trials. The test was just a machine moving over my body and was over in a very short time. The people in the testing area were all young and bright and I left there feeling positive. I would have to wait a couple of weeks for the results and then I will visit the oncologist again. Waiting for test results is never easy, but I seem to have done a lot of waiting since my first aspiration all those years ago.

It is surprising just how much of our heartbeat is silenced by our breast. Whenever I put my head on the pillow my heartbeat seems so much louder now without the cushioning of the breast. Breast cancer is in the news it seems almost every day and only this morning there was Kylie Minogue on the front page of the newspaper, newly diagnosed. Then there are the telephone calls, probably because people thought of me when they read the news item. 'I'd give anything for a little country cottage in the middle of a ten-acre paddock,' I say to Ian. People mean well, but I can do without these continual reminders of my mortality. Perhaps I should go to a support group where everyone is processing the same sort of information. I have resisted one because I could see myself empathising with everyone else's problems, and I have enough of my own.

Ian and I have decided to renovate the front garden. After over forty years in the house it needed a new look and the paths had been lifted in places – first by the gum trees we had planted and then later by the casuarinas. Autumn seems to have been particularly warm this year and there is still time to put in new plants before the winter. We go to the nursery and look at some camellias. I don't have time to wait for things to grow and so we choose three of a reasonable size. The workmen have already put down the concrete in readiness for pavers, the local council had removed all the street trees and are planting new ones next month, the firm has sent the wrong coloured pavers and they are stacked metres high on what remains of the nature strip. It has been weeks since the trees were removed and grubbed out and I am beginning to regret ever having thought of the idea, but Ian is reluctant to have help in the garden and once the new layout is complete there will be less lawn to be mowed and the garden beds can be managed without difficulty. It is a pity about the new lawn areas. It will be winter before they are down. I am thankful that we can afford the renovation but realised that of course we should have attended to all this years ago. But there had been so much crammed into our two lives and there never had been the time or the money earlier on.

There is a ruthlessness about living life to the full each day. The sitting room needs to be painted and although all the books will have to come out of the bookcases, and all the china and glassware from the sideboards, it is necessary if we are going to make cleaning easier for ourselves. I remove a whole lot of souvenirs and offer them to our sentimental eldest, the rest I take to the op shop. It is never easy to part with these things, but I feel that if I don't do it someone else will have to do it. That makes the task simpler, somehow. It is the same with my wardrobe. I am not good at discarding clothes, always thinking that the fashions will eventually come full circle. Of course they don't; the old clothes never seem quite right even if they are the right colour for the season. So out they went, filling two large plastic bags ready for the next clothes collection from whichever charity got in first.

I have friends who go through their wardrobe at the end of each season and cull. I envy them. I still have one or two things I could never quite part with. A long, black velvet princess-style gown I had worn to give out prizes at a school speech night, a beautiful blouse that I can no longer fit into and one or two other things that I think my granddaughter might like in a couple of years. Ian is just as bad. He has more 'gardening' jumpers than there are years left to garden in. I laugh as I go through the pile. There is, however, a corduroy jacket that one of my grandsons would just love, and they have certainly come back into fashion.

Clearing things out, sorting, freshening up the house. Psychologically it can all be explained, but I don't want to go there.

I read another one of Mary Oliver's poems from her collection *Why I Wake Early*. It says what I want to say:

Mindful

Every day
    I see or I hear
        something
            that more or less

kills me
    with delight,
        that leaves me
           like a needle

        in the haystack
           of light

The Kylie Minogue cancer story is all over the paper again. There are survivors' stories: television news programs telling of world-wide sympathy for her. Poor girl. As if it isn't enough to have to digest the news without dealing with the media as well. They mean well. They want to draw attention to the need for women to have regular breast examinations. But I know that even if you are very careful the thief can come in the night. There are diagrams showing milk ducts and lymph nodes and my oncologist is on television predicting a positive outcome for the celebrity patient. But as someone said and rightly, 'Once you're diagnosed with cancer, it never goes away.' You live ever after with the knowledge that one day it will return. In the meantime, there is each day to enjoy rather like a climber going up the slippery slope of a high mountain and not always having the courage to peer over the edge in case the sight prevents him taking another step. But I watch on television a woman truck driver negotiate the three-day journey through the mountains to La Paz. Three hundred people are killed on the narrow mountainous track every year, but the woman was strong, had a sense of humour and knew all the risks she was taking. *She* was courageous.

3

March

It was *Ladies in Lavender* that set my mind racing back to a little Cornish cove just like the deserted beach in the film. I can still see it vividly in my mind's eye. It was the early fifties and our first son, Peter, had a vivid yellow jumper, brown trousers and little red zippered boots. It was early spring and we had travelled down to Cornwall in our ancient Morris from the dormitory town of Crediton in Devon.

While we are driving home from *Ladies in Lavender* we talk of the superb performances of Judi Dench and Maggie Smith and of Truro, Mevagissey, Penzance, Land's End and Kynance Cove, where the photo of Peter had been taken. We both look so confident in the photo taken at Land's End, so confident that all would be well for our time in England. We had booked in at a bed and breakfast. A schoolmaster's salary didn't allow for extravagances. The landlady was an eccentric woman who seemed to spend a great deal of her time talking to her budgerigar. I inherited my aviphobia from my mother, I suspect, and was terrified that at any moment the bird would be let out of the cage while we were eating breakfast. We had packed so much into those five years away, so much into our life together.

I set about getting dinner. Preparing food is never a chore for me. It never has been, really, even in the early months of our marriage when confronted with an electric stove (we had gas at home) and with few culinary skills I had taken myself off to cooking lessons at the Electricity Trust of South Australia, where they did all sorts of things with dariol moulds, I think they were called. I like cooking meals for our friends. They always say that I fuss, but in fact I can prepare meals very quickly. I don't knit, don't sew, but cooking is a creative exercise for me. I can't make the delicate feather-like sponges my mother had made and then iced in such an expert way. The children still laughingly recall my famous butterfly sponges made into birthday cakes. I had perfected a chocolate sponge recipe that never failed and I have made it more times than I can remember. I don't have a sweet tooth, although I can remember that when I was teaching I would come into the house and look for chocolate to revive me in the late afternoon.

Shopping, especially for fruit and vegetables, gives me enormous pleasure. The greengrocers in the High Street is where I have shopped for over forty years. Of course it is ever so much bigger than it was in the sixties and is now being run by the children and grandchildren of the delightful Italian couple I remember. Only yesterday I bought chestnuts, two mangosteens (because I was fascinated by their delicate insides), sauce tomatoes, wonderful long, slender, sweet red peppers and a host of other vegetables. I often marvel at the variety of mushrooms and the sheer abundance of fruit and vegetables. In Devon, in the fifties, I was dismayed at the poor choice of vegetables, but they were all grown in and around the village and the fresh cabbage leaves ('spring greens' they were called) were often all that was available.

We had arrived in Devon after a four-week sea voyage with our baby son and after spending three months in Oak House in Putney. Oak House was an elegant Victorian home then serving as a small private hotel for elderly ladies or those who wanted to spend time at Wimbledon for the tennis. Peter was a greedy little chap and at breakfast each morning, Farquhar, who served as butler and handyman, would enquire whether I would 'take a little kipper'. I had wanted to say, 'I'll eat any number of kippers', such was my hunger, but I simply smiled politely. The elderly ladies already knew what they thought of these 'Orstralians' and I was determined not to give them any cause for complaint. Each week I would wheel our son in his low-slung Australian pram to be weighed and measured and each week I couldn't believe that he was still putting on eight ounces. Small wonder that I sometimes felt tired. He sucked strongly and would yell with hunger after his evening feed just as we had finished dinner. The elderly lady in the adjacent room would knock on the wall: Oak House was not accustomed to the sound of a baby crying. We found a car for ninety-eight pounds and although Ian was only earning ten pounds a week as a filing clerk we thought it was worth it. We would drive Peter in the back of the car around Richmond Park until he fell asleep then we would carry him very gingerly up the steep back stairs to our room where I would drink copious amounts of water before his ten o'clock feed.

For me it was a long summer. Each day Ian would go in to London to work, returning in time for dinner. Australian schoolmasters without connections to a school in the fifties had to try their luck against Oxford and Cambridge graduates and it didn't matter how good they were in the classroom. And who had heard of Adelaide or Melbourne as places of academic excellence?

I was grateful that my breasts were good milk machines. Before I left Australia, a health centre sister hat told me to drink a glass of Lactagol before each feed to keep up my milk supply. There was no such thing as demand feeding in the fifties. It mattered little whether you mixed it with water or milk, it always tasted like fine sand. Occasionally when I complained, Ian would say, 'It can't be that bad, dear.' One evening I said rather testily, 'You have a taste, then.' 'Horrible' was his verdict, and I felt much better.

Peter was born in Adelaide on a hot February night while fires raged in the Adelaide hills. I had been in labour some hours before the taxi driver, at great speed, had taken Ian and me to the hospital in the early hours of the morning. In those days we had a motorbike and sidecar – hardly the way to travel to a hospital! I slept through most of the day, Ian had visited me in the evening and had been so gentle in his concern. Then, after he left the labour room, maybe as a result of his tenderness, quite suddenly my legs were up in stirrups and Peter came with a great rush and I felt torn apart by the speed of it all. Because my mother had insisted, I had a specialist for the pregnancy, but he had been called away to a difficult birth at another hospital and I was left in the theatre with the doctor on duty. Peter was seven pounds fourteen ounces, strong and healthy, but for several days I felt as though I was sitting on a barbed wire fence.

When the sister brought him in for his first feed, they took away his blanket so that I could examine him naked. Yes, he had the right number of fingers and toes, but in my innocence it had never occurred to me that he would not be complete. I put him to my breast and at that moment I had a sharp recollection of my mother sitting on the couch feeding my youngest brother. As I gingerly moved him towards my nipple the sister snapped, 'For goodness sake, hold him close.' I had felt so inadequate and immediately dissolved into tears. I was failing this precious child.

We soon discovered the mutual pleasure for both of us. He was a strong baby and gulped in so much air that he developed colic. After the two of us came home, when Ian came in from school I would thrust the pram at him and beg him to keep walking so that I could prepare the evening meal. We were living with Ian's widowed father and he had to be fed even if we could wait.

Three months later we were sailing for England in a tiny cabin on G deck. There were times when the ship heaved and shuddered and I would lie on the lower bunk as my son drained my breasts. The motion of the ship affected him and what went in seemed to come out the other end. He didn't gain any weight during those four long weeks. True, he didn't lose any, but all I had to do was eat and feed him. It should have been so easy with my head full of the intoxicating sights of Colombo, Bombay, Aden, Port Said and Malta.

After three months we went to the grammar school in Crediton and a boarding school house full of senior boys. When Ian had gone down for the interview, the headmaster had asked him if he was prepared to be in charge of a senior house they were converting for the senior boys. It had been the former school hospital, up the hill from the main school, and had been empty for some time. The gardener had used the entrance porch to place onions and bulbs in a dry place. As they came to view the house, the Head had pushed back the bulbs and assured Ian that it would all be tidied up before we came down after the summer holidays. In the event, nothing was done and we spent our first couple of weeks in the main school building in the San sleeping in narrow wrought-iron hospital beds. We made our flat in the house as comfortable as possible. We were determined to show these Englishmen that Australians had some style.

Painting the kitchen and feeding a growing boy was not always easy, but at nine months I stopped breast feeding and at ten months the energetic boy walked. The dormitories had highly polished floorboards and Peter would follow the housekeeper as she cleaned, tumbling over sometimes but getting up quickly with a giggle as if surprised that the floor could inflict pain.

Just before Easter, Ian's father died and my father, wanting to help in some way, sent enough money for us to have an Easter break. We decided to go to Denmark to see if Ian had any relatives there. But with a name as common as Smith or Jones… The Danes were so welcoming even though we relied on our dictionary much of the time. By now my breasts had returned to their normal size. A bit of a shame, I thought. Ian had appreciated their larger size and we laughed about it.

While in Copenhagen we took the Oslo to Bergen rail journey in the company of two Americans whose three sons were at home and into their teens. The Americans didn't seem to mind this energetic child clambering all over them for the long day's journey. The train was full of families going to the snowfields and at each stop they saw tiny red-clad figures with their own tiny skis. Ian and I liked the Norwegians, we discovered. It wasn't just the beautiful landscape we enjoyed; it was the fresh and open way they engaged with tourists. Nothing seemed too much trouble for them.

We came home with so many pictures in our heads, of exotic sculptures in Frogner Park in Oslo, the extraordinary murals in the town hall, the Danish fishwives, windows full of smorrebrod, those tastefully arranged open sandwiches, the ancient capital at Roskilde, stylish furniture that was replicated in the attractive flats, storks nesting on top of buildings, the shining beauty of the fjords, the Little Mermaid statue, the cobbled streets, the bicycles, and the extraordinary tower of the Bourse, the beautiful stainless steel and the style of the Danes.

The Devon school appointment was for one year only and it was necessary to stay in the south of England so that Ian could complete his Master's Degree in Education at Southampton University. He was able to find a position at the Portsmouth Northern Grammar School for Boys and I had seen an agency advertised in the *Daily Telegraph* called En Famille where families exchanged homes with European families. The agency said it didn't have to be an exchange. We could stay with an Austrian family, and they supplied three photos of different homes. We chose Gotzis near the provincial capital, Feldkirch. The young couple had a daughter the same age as our Peter and welcomed us to their home. It looked like every Austrian home one could imagine with window boxes full of begonias, a splendid vegetable garden tended by the mother, Claudi, and from the top of the gentle rise at the back of the house an incredible view over the valley of the Rhone with the mountains a glorious backdrop.

Returning thirteen years later with our now three children, we found the quiet simple, rural hamlet had become a hive of industrial activity with motorways and speeding traffic. Perhaps part of this complex journey of life is the way we deal with change, adapting to it and somehow gaining strength from the new experiences. I discovered that it is never wise to return to places that have given us special memories. All too often they have changed over the years and we wish we had never returned.

Before long, the Hansen family had exchanged the tranquil beauty of Devon for a dockyard city. There were enticing places only a short distance away but the terrace houses were dark and uninviting and had changed little since the end of the war, when Portsmouth had been so heavily bombed. But there were compensations. The neighbours, who saw Australians as something of a novelty, smiled often, and I made some good friends.

We didn't wait too long between children, and in any case this was before the days of the contraceptive pill and families did not always turn out as planned. I became pregnant again and this time without the morning sickness I had with Peter. But like the gall wasps, all pregnancies are different. At three months it seemed that I would lose this new living creature within me. The doctor on weekend duty said to me, 'You might as well get up. You'll probably lose it anyway.' My own GP, who had spent some time in Australia and seemed to understand our isolation, told me that if I was prepared to stay in bed for a couple of weeks I might just be able to carry this baby to full term. Anything, I thought. Anything. So each morning Ian would drop Peter off at a neighbour's house in the next street and go off to the grammar school while I lay all day on the downstairs on the couch in the bleak, grey house in the bleak, grey city, and prayed for a miracle. I wrote letters home regularly full of cheerful news. They didn't need to know of my discomfort, and my mother already found the twelve thousand miles difficult.

When I finally was told I could get up, I couldn't believe that the tiny thing within me might be all right. All that blood loss. Could everything be as the doctor said? For the remainder of the pregnancy I lived with both hope and fear. I had to believe that this now quickened child would be whole.

The house we rented from an elderly woman who had gone into a nursing home. There were rugs to cover carpets and mats to cover the rugs and antimacassars to cover the lounge suite. The only heat came from the small gas fire in the sitting room. Not much comfort when there was a fall of snow, but Peter and I would stand at the window marvelling at the snowflakes as they fell. This didn't happen very often because Portsmouth was close to the sea, but when it did snow it transformed the depressing streets and little gardens. Now I was six months pregnant, walking to the shops a hazardous affair and I would beg Peter not to run ahead.

The first week of May with rhododendrons, azaleas, trees drowning in fresh greenness we took a Sunday afternoon drive out into the Hampshire countryside. Peter fell asleep in the back of the car and not wanting to disturb the peace and quiet we kept driving. It was such a glorious spring day.

After dinner I felt strangely energetic and decided to do the ironing before I went up to bed. Ian said, 'Aren't you tired? It has been a long day.' But I didn't feel tired at all. Peter had been bathed, had his dinner and was fast asleep. These were the treasured moments of the day for Ian and for me. He could work on his thesis, I could read, iron, write letters or type Ian's next chapter. We went up to bed, passing on the walls *The Monarch of the Glen* and *Heavenwards*, those hideous Victorian reproductions beloved by a particular generation. I found them all too depressing but kept on reminding myself that this was not for ever. I checked on Peter as we passed his room. He was fast asleep.

A few hours later I was woken up by strong contractions. My doctor had said that it might be a quick birth this time and I didn't know whether to wake Ian or lie there for a bit. Teaching in the dockyard city was very demanding and he needed all the sleep he could get. Before long the contractions were too strong and I woke Ian up. It was three o'clock in the morning and we couldn't wake anyone at that hour to come and stay with Peter. I prayed that Peter wouldn't wake up while Ian took me to the nursing home. It was a quick journey at that time of night to Eddystone, named after the famous lighthouse. I had met the matron several months before when I made the booking to have my baby there. At that time in England you could only have your first baby in hospital but with no family nearby my doctor thought it best for me to go to the nursing home. His own home was just behind the hospital so he could be there in a short time if necessary. It seemed ages before a sister, her hair still in rollers, answered the doorbell. She said she had a patient in labour and told Ian to go back home to our son. I stood in the hall waiting for the sister to return and a warm tabby cat came brushing up against me. It all seemed very domestic and when the sister came back it was to take me upstairs and tell me to get into my bed and she would be up shortly. There were two sleeping women in the other beds and I knew the contractions were too strong to keep quiet. I rang the bell and asked if I might go into the labour room. The sister replied she was sure my baby wouldn't arrive for a while and in any case she had a woman in advanced labour downstairs, but if I insisted I could go into the labour room. If the arrival of the baby was still some time away, I wondered how much stronger the contractions could get. Suddenly there was a strange feeling between my legs. I put my hand down and felt the baby's head. Leaning on the bell, I left my hand there until the sister arrived. 'Goodness me. The baby's almost here. There's no point in calling Doctor Mason now. You have a baby son.' He was eight pounds six ounces with a head covered with black hair. Later when he opened his eyes I couldn't believe it but they were brown.

In some ways it was almost like a home birth. When the morning staff came on, they carried me downstairs and David, our new son, was placed in the bassinet at the foot of my bed. The other two women in the room were warm and welcoming. When visitors came to see the other two women, they would peep into David's cot out of politeness, and the first thing they all said was 'What a lot of hair he has.' I thought he was beautiful.

It was the gall wasp again. No two exactly alike. David just ate and slept. When he latched on to my breast he would suck energetically on one side and then fall asleep. I knew I could wake him up for the other breast but he always looked so replete. Why was he such a good baby? Could the threatened miscarriage have done more damage than they had imagined? Was he slow? Retarded? But I had other things to occupy my mind with. While I was still in hospital Ian broke his arm trying to save a little girl from a fall in the playground near the hospital where he and Peter went each afternoon before visiting me. He only had one good arm, really. Polio had damaged his right side and this was his good left arm. I sometimes wonder how I managed, where I found the strength, the sheer physical energy to feed the baby and amuse his energetic young brother, and all this without a car, a dishwasher, a washing machine, or a deep freeze. Often in the following winter the nappies (no disposable ones then) would be frozen on the line overnight. Peter was very protective of his younger brother and since he spent most of his time eating and sleeping Peter thought he wasn't much trouble really. Mummy still had time to play with him and he liked shopping with David now sitting up in the pram looking at everything.

I was often homesick. Australian visitors to Portsmouth were rare. It was not on the tourist route really, and in any case most of the travelling overseas was being done by couples without young children. Only Nelson's *Victory* enticed them to Portsmouth. Ian was busy with his thesis on the rise of English in the secondary school curriculum. We had purchased an Olivetti typewriter in Aden on the way over and it was put to good use. Twice a month we would put the boys in the car and drive to Southampton. After Ian's morning visit we would have a picnic lunch at places like Winchester, or the New Forest, Buckler's Hard or Beaulieu Abbey. We wanted to make the most of every opportunity to see the countryside.

Ian needed to spend time in Oxford and kind friends offered us their home while they were on holiday. It was within easy reach of Oxford and seemed an ideal summer break. Ian had decided that he would forget about his research for a day and we would all have a day together at Blenheim Palace. It promised to be a beautiful summer's day. Our little Morris was maroon and blue. On reflection, white or yellow might have served us better. As we drew level with the Indian Institute in Oxford, a large truck carrying tubular steel and coming against the lights ploughed into the side of the car as it took the corner. Peter had been sitting on my lap (it was long before the days of seatbelts) and David was in the top of his pram in the back seat. I was bleeding profusely above the eye, Ian was bruised and Peter unable to take it all in. The shock prevented me from speaking and before long

I was rushed by ambulance to the Radcliffe Infirmary. It was time for David's feed and my breasts were full to overflowing. A New Zealand doctor assured me that I would be stitched up in no time and that there wouldn't be a bad scar. What I wanted to say was 'What about my breasts, my milk? Is this going to affect my supply?' I was young and shy and didn't want to bother him with my other problems. The sooner I could get back to Ian and the children the better.

We hired a car at the end of our stay in Aylesbury to take us back to Portsmouth but it was several months before the insurance company had sorted out the claim for our car and we were able to buy another. But my breasts didn't dry out – evidently a possibility after severe shock – and my younger son thrived. I was able to feed him for nine months.

Ian's final teaching appointment was in London. I had a marvellous time at Eltham College. The boys loved Ian and he loved the boys. But for the distance, those twelve thousand miles, we could have stayed there forever. In our third-floor flat in the former headmaster's house I could see Ian coming across for lunch each day, and the staff in the other two flats of the house were so agreeable. The master in the flat below was the school's music master and he and I often played duets together. I missed my piano so much and he told me one afternoon that his dentist wanted to move a grand piano from his home and thought he might like it. 'So I've decided the rosewood would make great coffee tables.' I blush even now when I remember my shocked response. 'You couldn't do that to a piano.' 'I hadn't thought,' he said, 'but perhaps you might care to have it.' I couldn't believe my ears. Two unnervingly small men had carried it up the two flights of stairs and there wasn't a mark on it as they placed it in the sitting room. I couldn't believe my good fortune.

On the ground floor lived the school chaplain and his two daughters, just a little younger than our two boys. Each afternoon we would go for walks around the nearby little tarn with its romantic trees. I never tired of it and the children enjoyed each other's company. All six of the adults in the house got on well. We were all so different temperamentally. That summer Ian was awarded his Master's degree by the Duke of Wellington and it was a grand occasion with candidates kneeling to have their hoods placed on them. Ian had participated fully in the life of Eltham, coaching athletics, enjoying his English teaching. It would be so much easier these days with phonecalls so cheap and travel so easy, but we were homesick.

After five years away we took our two boys home. Again by sea. It was too expensive to fly and we were thankful for the space allowed for our furniture which we had accumulated in the time we were in England. The ports held their usual fascination and it was such a luxury not to have to prepare meals for the boys. Of course we went down to the nursery at meal times just to make sure the boys ate well and we spent a great deal of the voyage in company with other Australian professionals returning from overseas study with their young children. We talked of our time in England as we sat on the children's deck watching over our small ones. I knew I had changed while away. I had left Australia a young, timid girl and I was returning a more confident woman who felt able to manage most situations, or so I thought.

The years away had been good years, and I had made some wonderful friends. I had enjoyed the two boarding schools. I liked the teenage boys, their openness, their ready acceptance of our young sons. Everyone had been so obliging. I remembered how in Crediton for our first English Christmas I had wanted to give the boys in our house a party before the end of term and I had casually remarked that it would be nice to liven up the appearance of the dormitory with some holly. I had noticed the big fat berries on the hedges as I walked Peter in his pram. It was a Sunday afternoon and usually the boys went for a walk out into the nearby countryside. Later that afternoon there was a knock at the back door and several of the boys were standing there, their arms bearing enormous great branches of holly. 'Will these do?' they asked. I remember that party so vividly. Ian and I had gone to the town's cakeshop and bought all the cakes so loved by teenage boys and the tables groaned with food.

Ian had enjoyed his school duties. He had taken a group of boys on a camping excursion to Dartmoor, had taken boys from Portsmouth up to London to see their first Shakespearean play, cycled around Belgium with senior scouts and gone to Germany with school cadets.

Returning home, we had hoped for a boarding school post but Ian was an Adelaidian and didn't have a Melbourne network. Eventually after three months of supply teaching we were given the senior boarding house position at Haileybury, with three charming housemasters and seventy boys, mostly from the country.

Although Peter was not yet five, the headmaster agreed to let him begin school. He could walk out the back gate to the school's primary section and he was deliriously happy. David, ever the dreamer, would play happily, amusing himself until Peter came in from school. The housemaster's house was right in the middle of the school and there were times as I pegged out the washing in full view of the bursar's office and the bookroom staff I felt as if I was in a goldfish bowl, but there were so many compensations.

Surrounded by school noise and bells, I couldn't have been happier. One of the housemasters was a movie buff and set up one of the games rooms in the boarding house as a cinema most Saturday evenings to entertain the boys. The staff had proper theatre seats brought in for the occasion, there were curtains that moved back before the national anthem was played and it was all great fun. It didn't seem to matter that the rooms of the housemaster's house were small and the laundry floor so uneven that I had to make do with its copper and wringer; it was certainly better than the copper and old mangle in Portsmouth. We purchased a small twin-tub washing machine that we could move across the floor in the one large space in the house – a kitchen cum dining area. I couldn't believe how easy it all was now or how quickly the clothes dried after the very fast spin dryer. I accompanied the school production of *HMS Pinafore* and enjoyed every moment. Life was good.

We had always thought a big family would be nice. Ian was an only child but I had grown up with three younger brothers and knew what family life could be like. With seventy boys around me, I didn't fancy my chances of having a daughter but it didn't really matter too much to me so long as the baby was healthy. Becoming pregnant had never been difficult for me and it wasn't long before the school doctor, who was my GP, was telling me that yes, I was pregnant, as I had thought.

Fortunately I was well through the pregnancy and the country boys saw birth as a fact of life, so as I grew they rarely seemed to notice. In 1962 women still tended to cover up any signs of pregnancy in the early months but the boarders' parents would enquire about my health whenever they visited the school. The Easter break was late that year and the family had all enjoyed the days off when the school was unusually quiet. The boys returned on the Tuesday evening and we had made arrangements with one of the housemasters that should the baby come at night he would keep an eye on the boys. My waters broke and I thought it was time to move to the hospital. Ian hadn't been present for the two other births and I was determined that this time he would have the pleasure of seeing his child born. He stayed in the room with me until a nursing sister said that she thought the birth would not be for some time. The baby's head was turned and unless forceps were used it would take a little time. The GP came and went and the sister sponged my forehead. I thought that labour would go on for ever but at one o'clock our daughter came into the world weighing seven pounds thirteen ounces. When the doctor told me I had a daughter I couldn't believe it and in the days following the birth I kept smiling whenever I looked at the dainty creature lying in my arms.

My breasts supplied all the milk my daughter needed, but from the very beginning she was not the hungry child the boys had been. She seemed satisfied with little, continuing to gain in weight, but the gains were nothing like the boys. I supposed that girls were just different feeders.

The day Jane was born, the boarding house boys and staff were delighted that there would be a girl in the house and on the flagpole was hoisted a large pink ribbon announcing her arrival. There were bunny rugs, dainty jackets and all manner of feminine gifts and dozens of cards. I knew now what my mother had meant when she had said, many years before, that if you have three children you might as well have six, it is the third that makes the family. And she was right. It required patience from both Peter and David, who had become accustomed to having all my attention, but they fussed over their little sister and were happy to stand by the pram and amuse her as she got older. But her feeding was still a problem. In desperation I would express my milk and try to feed her with a spoon, but nothing seemed to work. The health centre sister castigated me as though I alone was responsible for the paltry three or occasionally four ounces she gained each week.

I was so busy in the afternoons when the day staff left. The telephone would ring, usually just when I had the two boys in the bath and Jane was restless before her next feed. A mother would enquire whether her son had left his cap on the oval, or could she find out whether a boy had left the school grounds for home as she was running late to pick him up. And so it went. My mother thought that perhaps if I had a week at home away from the hustle and bustle of the school it might be better for both me and the baby. I hated leaving Ian and the boys but it seemed the only thing left to try. At five months it was decided that I should put Jane onto a bottle and SM33 was a formula recommended. We all discovered that she took comparatively little even from the bottle. She was a healthy baby, progressing well, but with a dainty appetite. I felt that I had failed in those early months but finally came to the realisation that all children are individuals from the moment of their birth.

For me, being a mother and a housemaster's wife was all that I needed to feel fulfilled. Today it might be said that I had given up my own career for the sake of my husband. But it wasn't like that at all in the early sixties for most women. Unless they were a single parent or were able to afford home help, their careers were either put on hold or in some cases never taken up again, although the skills were not forgotten.

One evening towards the end of our second year there was a telephone call from a member of the Melbourne University's Education Faculty inviting Ian to come up to the university to talk to them. He thought it was to be a conversation about a higher degree he was thinking of. To his astonishment he was offered a lectureship. What were we going to do? Peter, who had travelled the world with us, was now happy and settled in school. We were all happy and settled. But I knew Ian's capabilities. I knew that he needed a wider audience, for he was a born teacher. We had very little money in the bank. What we had had been spent on a new station wagon because we knew we would be taking boarders here and there and it had plenty of room. But moving! I couldn't bear the thought of it. Jane was not yet walking and here we were rushing up from Brighton to look at houses in suburbs within easy reach of schools and the university. I had worked so hard at making our half-house at Haileybury into a pleasant home. I loved the coming and going of boys, the sheer energy of the place. But I knew I would adjust to change in due course.

On a hot, mid-week afternoon we were shown a house whose design had come out of Walter Burley Griffin's office. We were desperate to find somewhere before we had to leave the school, and the idea of a home of our own was bliss. The house was rather masculine in design, I thought, and the painting of it left a lot to be desired, but I thought of our other flats and decided that it had possibilities. Especially when we went inside. The ceilings were high, the house cool, and the university would take on the mortgage of the house if they found the property to be sound. Built in the 1920s, its construction was solid, and the loan went through.

The only way we could afford the repayments and at the same time independent school fees for Peter was to have two student boarders. There were two upstairs rooms and I was sure I could manage. It was rather like having five children, but at least Peter would be in a happy environment and he had been our chief concern.

'No more moves,' I had said when we settled into Haileybury. Now, more than forty years on and still in the same house, I realise that our life has been too crammed to ever think of looking at houses and the thought of another move horrified Ian. We would stay here, I thought, until the upkeep became too much for us to manage.

4

May

I saw the oncologist today. He is warm, a good listener, and he left me feeling that I could depend on him in any eventuality.

'You have beautiful bones,' he said, and I laughed, thinking to myself of all the milk I used to drink in my teens. I have never liked tea and it was only after my marriage that I began to drink coffee and came to enjoy it. Now all the milk and milkshakes had left me with 'beautiful bones'. This now gave me the option of Arimidex as an alternative hormone therapy to Tamoxifen. The survival rate for someone with an affected lymph node, even if only one, was slightly better, it appeared, on Arimidex in my case. All medications have some side effects and those I had experienced from Tamoxifen had been comparatively minor so we had a fall-back position if I couldn't cope with the new drug.

These choices that need to be made during any illness are difficult. All you can do is weigh up the evidence and trust that it will work for you. It was the wretched gall wasp again. We are all unique, all different. While I see this as miraculous, there are times when I think it may have made life simpler if we were all the same.

Sitting in the waiting room with women about to have chemotherapy or frail aged with advanced illness, I find it easier to make conversation with the woman next to me rather than stare into space as so many do, or flip through a magazine. The woman next to me is a sprightly eighty-year-old who is accompanying her daughter to the specialist. The eighty-year-old has never had a mammogram and yet here is her daughter in her forties having chemotherapy for breast cancer.

As we chat, I am reminded of the French film Ian and I saw the day before. *A Common Thread*. I think it might remain one of my favourite films along with *Babette's Feast, Rain Man, Portrait of a Lady, Jesus of Montreal, Gabbeh, Gallipoli* and *The Weeping Camel*. The film tells the story of a pregnant seventeen-year-old who comes to work for an embroiderer who does work for Parisian couturiers. The woman's son had been killed in an accident and she was still grief-stricken; the girl's unwanted pregnancy was becoming more obvious as the weeks passed. The two women find a common thread in their ability to embroider what become exquisite pieces of fabric. Their adversity seems to bring them closer together as does the work the young girl is able to do under the guidance of Madame Melikian. The threads of their embroidery serve as a metaphor for their life threads. There is the click of needles as their hands glide through the gossamer-fine material, and as the work proceeds so does their relationship. It seems as though there is a bond between women when they meet at vulnerable points in their lives, childbirth, a child's first day at school, weddings, deaths. The bond often happens quite quickly and has very little to do with age or race.

In an oncologist's waiting room there is no time for conversation about the weather or matters of little importance in the larger scheme of things. Perhaps it was the concern on the woman's face that caused me to begin the conversation. Here was a mother concerned for her daughter and wishing that she could take her place. I can remember saying to a friend many years before that we should all have to visit a hospital waiting room for a reality check when we become preoccupied with the superficial things of life.

I have my first tablet the following night. It was to be only every second day for the first three weeks. I feel tired the next day and decide that it is just imagination. I have a telephone call from someone from the ABC's *Life Matters* program asking permission to publish the love letter Ian had given me in hospital. When Ian had had his autobiography *The Naked Fish* published, I had felt very vulnerable, but then all the letters started coming from people who had appreciated his honesty and openness and I had to forget about my own timidity. Perhaps my writing might be of interest to others, too. People were always asking when I was going to write my autobiography, and so I thought I should at least try, if only to set it down for the grandchildren. There was also the possibility that it might be an encouragement for others with breast cancer.

In a radio interview, Michael Biwater, a Cambridge classicist, said that 'we are defined by what we have lost'. It set me thinking again about loss, for the loss of my breast was nothing compared with the loss of people who had been part of my life. I remembered the sudden loss of my mother, who died the night before she was to be admitted to hospital for treatment for her heart condition. My mother had seen the specialist that afternoon and, with that strange premonition that some people have, seemed certain that although she was only in her early sixties her life was finished. Early the following morning my father telephoned to say that my mother had died after being taken by ambulance to the hospital during the night.

Of course when I heard the news I went through the motions of organising the children off to school and then began to help my father and brothers plan the funeral. I am the eldest and the only girl and I knew what was expected of me, but I wanted the world to stop. How dare everyone go on as if nothing had happened! I moved through the next few days in a fog of deep grief, numb to everything around me but able to prepare food for friends coming back after the funeral. There was a look of total devastation on my father's face and I couldn't look into my brothers' eyes.

My father later remarried and lived to celebrate his ninetieth birthday in fine style with his children, grandchildren and great-grandchildren. When at the age of ninety-four he was admitted to hospital, my stepmother was also in another hospital so I was able to spend the weeks before he died with him. He had only spent one day in hospital during his long life and, although I knew that he needed to be there, I knew he hated hospitals. When he was growing up, if you went to hospital you died there. You didn't come home. Now he had a fatal blood disease and I was sure he knew that he was not going home.

People keep saying that time is a great healer, but I also know that for many people that just isn't true. As you get older you come to accept that great grief is the price we pay for great love and loving and loss sit together.

I can hear in my mind's ears the sound of my father's voice even now. It was like all the Welsh tenors I had ever listened to, strong and sweet. He had often told us about his father, who had died when Dad was only six, and of the beautiful singing voice he had. How good it will be, I thought, for this current generation who can preserve not only a host of visual images, but also the voices of those they love. I have often wished that I could hear my mother's voice as clearly as my father's, but thirty-five years have passed and they have dulled the sound in my memory.

Michael Biwater had said that 'all that we have had glows more brightly'. I want to hold on to all that brightness. There has been so much of it.

I was reading a book review. It was about Michael Winter's latest book, *The Big Why*. At one point in the book he had written,

> The question is not were you loved. Or did you love. Or did you love yourself. Or did you allow love to move you, though that's a big one. Move you.
> The question, Rockwell, is did you get to be who you are. And if not then why. That, my friend, is the big why.

I suppose, I thought, that we go on discovering more and more about who we are all through life. Who we are in so many different circumstances. There were always more revelations.

I hadn't ever looked far enough ahead to think about a life-threatening illness confronting me. It is there for all of us eventually and certainly after my seventieth birthday I had decided that every year after my three score years and ten would be a bonus year. But even with all my aspirated cysts over so many years I felt sure that since I was having regular check-ups I would probably end my days as my mother had, of a heart condition.

I was discovering that any illness that is life-threatening takes us on a journey that we have to take alone, or, if we believe, with God. Even when surrounded by those who love us, we ask the question, 'Who am I now that all this confronts me?' What is it at the core of my being that will enable me to be thankful for the gift of each new day? I have always loved the words of Joyce Grenfell in one of her books, 'God is not a think, he's a feel.' I have wrestled with God-talk most of my life and now find that understanding God at depth is for me every bit as much to do with the senses as the mind.

Teaching my Year 12 classes in the 1980s, when girls often resisted anything other than exam work, made me determined to help them think about the meaning of life. Jack Priestley from Exeter University had written about education for both our inner and outer worlds. In an article he had quoted from Navonne, 'Man lives in two worlds and when he tries to live in just one something seems to go wrong with him.'

In the early years of schooling, the two worlds are almost equal with the inner world of the imagination, emotions and subjectivity, but in the secondary years we concentrate more and more on the world of material facts. Education has to lead to a job, education is no longer seen as a preparation for living.

Body and mind we are good at, but spirit we neglect. I wanted the girls I taught, who would one day be doctors, nurses, lawyers, teachers and parliamentarians, and engaged in an enormous variety of careers, to think about what it means to live well, so that everything they became involved in would be set against a value system that they had wrestled with for themselves as individuals. We often had some fiery discussions in my classes, but most of the time I left the classroom feeling that what I was attempting to do was worthwhile.

5

Ian had finished his doctorate and we were ready in 1969 for a sabbatical year in London and Cambridge. The three children, now thirteen, eleven and seven, were full of anticipation. Of course there would still be school, but there was the romance of a long sea voyage before that. It was cheaper still to travel overseas by sea, and I was glad that luggage would not be a problem. Today, with cruising so fashionable and when there are liners of unimaginable luxury, I thought of our cabins. After the awful experience on G deck in the 1950s I thought our accommodation positively luxurious, and the thought of us all enjoying Perth, Durban, Cape Town, Dacca and Lisbon was wonderful. I knew how much we would revel in the exotic sight and smells of each port and the lasting impression it would make on us. As I prepared the house for the young couple who would be occupying it while we were away, I told myself the effort was worth it.

Having a sabbatical leave together had required savings of all kinds during the previous six years and the children knew that a great deal of their summer holiday time would be taken up with their father marking unending public exam English papers in the hot study, only appearing for a cool drink or at meal times. When I think back on this period of our lives I wonder whether the children saw us play enough. Ian's doctorate had to be researched and written mostly in his own time and I found myself telling the children not to go up to the study unless they really had to.

We rented a television set only during school holidays. Ian wanted them to become avid readers, which they did, but they liked nothing better on a hot day than to sit and watch a favourite program together. It would be so different today.

The three children had always got on well together. The boys were so different temperamentally and they had always protected their younger sister so that when it came to meal times on board ship we rarely had to stay very long in the dining room with them and in the evening there was the great luxury of dressing for dinner and eating with friends. There was something about four weeks at sea that helped you adjust to a different part of the world. You felt something for the long sea voyages of explorers who had often not seen land for weeks on end. Each port visited could be digested by the children before the next, and so their memories have stayed with them.

In 1977 we had another sabbatical. So much had happened since 1969. My mother had died in 1970, my father had remarried, our elder son had left university and a Commonwealth scholarship in favour of jackerooing and then a Farm Management course. Our second son had a scholarship to a university college and our daughter was still at secondary school.

Just five weeks before we left for overseas I had gone to see a specialist who after examining me said bluntly, 'Are you going to have a hysterectomy now or shall I give you the name of a London surgeon?' Of course I wanted to have it in my own city and so we had flown to Greece, going overland so that David and Jane could experience Athens, Venice, Salzburg, Vienna and Paris on our way to Cambridge. Peter would be in Queensland on a cattle property for the whole year before his final year at college and I knew that I would worry with him out of easy contact, but this was the 'letting go' that writers keep on telling us about.

We rented a house in the little village of Coton, in those days just a cycle track's distance from the university. In 1969 we had rented a house in Barton from a now world-famous astronomer, Dr Chandra Wickramasinghe.

Barton was only a short distance from Coton and the two villages were very much alike. Time seemed to stand still. Both had the village church and the school at their centre and the village store where everyone was known and where the arrival of an Australian family was an event to be noticed.

A simple shopping expedition into Cambridge along the Grantchester Road was a delight with the neat hedges, ploughed fields and nearby college towers. Jane and David had remembered the famous Fitzbilly buns from our last time in Cambridge and they were as delicious as we had remembered them. I loved the market square with its stalls of cheese or fish or flowers or tempting second-hand books. We never failed to make the most of evensong at St John's or Kings. In winter there were very few tourists about but the student calendar was full of interesting events. In late January there was an exhibition of David Hockney prints and a graduation at the Senate House. The men wore white bow ties and clerical bands with their ermine-trimmed gowns and the women were in dark skirts with white blouses. Proud parents were everywhere taking photos. Cambridge is unlike Oxford in many ways. The university and the town seem melded together with open fields and the fen countryside surrounding the town. It was like living in a dish of rich cream. There was a sculptor in the village living in an Elizabethan house opposite the rectory. If only we could have afforded to buy one of her pieces.

Ian had two projects for his leave. The first was to write a book for English teachers and as well he had a regular column to produce for Melbourne's *Education Age*. This of course meant that everyone knew where we were living and we had an endless flow of Australian visitors for most of the year. Jane did her schoolwork by correspondence and David did cleaning at one of the colleges and audited a Fine Arts course at the university. He decided to do his honours thesis on the west front of Peterborough Cathedral, so there were lots of visits to Peterborough. Ian was a Visiting Fellow of Wolfson College and had been given a room in the Education Department where he could write undisturbed.

We frequently walked or drove to nearby villages. In Hauxton there was a church established from the cathedral at Ely in AD 700 with a gorgeous wall painting of Thomas a'Beckett. David became fascinated by the church brasses. Today many of them have been removed but in the 1970s you could wander in and rub them to your heart's content.

In early February we had our first fall of snow and I watched while the small children next door made a snowman and I went walking around the village just to see the beauty of the church and fallow fields covered with their white blanket.

It is so cold here in Melbourne this morning. Our first really cold morning since last September and we are already in June. We have had more fogs than usual but when they lift we get sunny afternoons. The weather reminds me of winter mornings in Cambridge when we woke to find that the boiler had gone out during the night and since it was the only form of heating we had there were rapid attempts made by Ian and David to get it going again. I remembered the winter weather in Devon when the kitchen cum living room was filled with smoke from the stove that was supposed to provide both heating and cooking facilities. We had tried to get it going and on New Year's Eve had sat huddled around its small flames to listen to the world premiere of Dylan Thomas's *Under Milk Wood*. I can never hear it read without being transported back to Devon. The general consensus was that being 'Orstralian' we could manage and eventually we were given a school griller with a hotplate capable of taking two saucepans. There were some great people on the staff and one family had us home every Sunday for a roast dinner. Such kindness we will never forget. In 1960 in London in our third-floor flat we had only a minute gas fire and had bought a convection heater which because of the low ceilings adequately heated the living area.

Most nights after the boys were asleep Ian worked at his thesis while I typed it up. The couch was a wartime sofa bed which we had to assemble when our evening work was completed. Exhaustion tends to make you forget the hardest of mattresses. I loved the flat and the only drawback was hauling washing downstairs accompanied by two active little boys and if I left them in the garden to play I had to watch from the window that they didn't leave the garden. There was no side gate.

What is it about extremes of temperature that triggers memories?

The cold reminds me of our visit to George Steiner in Geneva. When we asked him where we might spend a few days before Ian's work began in Venice, he suggested Chamonix. We had arrived at the station on a bitterly cold cloudy day with not a mountain in sight and the pavement so slippery with ice that it made getting cases to the hotel more than a little difficult. Hotel rooms are probably not so very different if you stay in the four- or five-star variety but lower down the scale they have so much character. The room in Chamonix was so very French, period chairs and table, dainty wallpaper and matching bedspread and curtains. There were two little wrought-iron balconies opening off the room but with the dense fog outside you could see no further than the houses on the opposite side of the street.

The following morning Ian called me to the balcony and opened the window. The fog had lifted, there was bright sunshine and it seemed as if the mountain peaks of the Mont Blanc range were hanging over the town. We took the train to the Mer de Glace that afternoon. It looked like a sea of ice tossed by a storm and it possessed that extraordinary glacial blue that is indescribable.

The next morning we took the cable car to the top of one of the peaks and sat in the hot sun with the snow sparkling like diamonds. Hang gliders were preparing their run off to the valley below, where church bells were calling, people were out in the streets buying exotic cakes in decorated boxes, and others were carrying fresh baguettes under their arm. Ruskin's Walk was a steep climb up a slope to a dense pine forest and then marvellous views of the mountains.

In our seven years of living overseas we had never experienced a white Christmas, but en route to Venice we had gone for Christmas to Anif, two kilometres from Salzburg, staying at the large and very comfortable Hotel Friesacher. After booking in we went for a walk around the village just as the sun was setting pale pink behind the mountains. A heavy fall the previous week had left snow piled high on the side of the roads and the castle at Anif was like something from a fairytale with its frozen lake and moat, a thin sliver of a moon, ducks and swans huddled beneath the trees that seemed dark and mysterious against the fading light of the sky.

We had woken up to snow the following morning and it continued snowing for several days, to the delight of all the visitors. In Salzburg the Cathedral Square was crowded with stalls selling freshly cut Christmas trees. There were singers singing carols while Father Christmas was busy bringing children into the square in a horse-drawn wagon. Opposite the main entrance to the cathedral was the traditional market selling tree decorations. The Austrians seem to have perfected the art of Christmas celebration and decoration. Christmas Eve was heralded with booming bells from the cathedral where the high altar was ablaze with candles and decorated with bowls of red poinsettias and gold ribbons. There were ten Christmas trees in various parts of the cathedral. The Haydn Mass with choir and orchestra and the procession of clergy in their richly embroidered vestments was memorable, but on Christmas morning we heard a Mozart Mass and it seemed as if the choir's voices had been made to sing Mozart.

On Christmas night Ian and I were taken by friends to dinner in a restaurant at Kuchl, a little village not far from Anif. The streets were thick with snow and lights were strung across the streets like necklaces. The restaurant was adjacent to a floodlit onion-spired church and inside the warmth came from the great blue china heater in one corner of the room. Austrians have good appetites and their meal was festive with smoked salmon followed by enormous platters of chicken and veal accompanied by fruit and vegetables.

In Salzburg, I had delighted in our visit to the world famous Marionette theatre, where inanimate puppets were transformed into the fluid movements of ballerinas in the traditional *Nutcracker Ballet*.

Memories are like slides in the mind. They can take us back in a second to a particular place and time. We often erase the difficult moments from the collection because they are too painful, but we retain the nourishing, nurturing ones to help us through difficult times.

6

I have been reading a long article on happiness. What is it? How do you define it? I had spent some time trying to define it. I decided that it mostly comes unbidden and usually when the senses are heightened, so that arranging a vase of flowers, preparing a meal, playing a Beethoven sonata or even just gazing out at a wintry sky with the bare branches of trees etched against the grey could bring me, for those few moments, utter delight.

Today I thought that happiness was my body's capacity, for this brief time certainly, to cope with the new drug regime. Arimidex hasn't been trialled as long as Tamoxifen, but the number of survivors is greater by something like six per cent.

Part of the problem with this illness is the necessity, at least in this early period, to see specialists regularly. You cannot just get on with life and forget all about it. I suppose that the longer I am on the medication the easier it will become.

I saw my surgeon for my three-month check-up this morning. He is rather shy and to compensate for his shyness I seem always to talk too much. I told him of the newspaper report from *The Lancet* which stated that ninety-four per cent of breast tumours in people at high risk of breast cancer – that is, with a family history of the disease – can be detected if there is a combination of both mammogram and MRI observations. He didn't comment and I was left wondering whether mine would have been picked up much earlier with MRI.

I read in the newspaper only today of a woman needing pain management after the removal of her lymph nodes during breast cancer surgery. I was thankful that apart from some stiffness under my arm I had very little discomfort from my surgery. The surgeon might be shy, I thought, but I was grateful for his skill.

I would need to have another mammogram on my remaining breast in October but at the moment things seemed to be going on satisfactorily way.

The most difficult aspect of the disease is its unpredictability. There is, however, a strange elation that is difficult to describe. At times I feel quite reckless about the things that are important, that need to be done. I want those things to have all of me, whatever the cost.

News items in the health section of the newspaper offered all sorts of optimism. The previous Saturday I had read a report which stated that Australian researchers 'have developed a new test that appears successful in detecting the site of hidden cancers, a possible breakthrough that should allow quicker treatment'. A cancer cell circulating in a patient's blood can be identified and studying its genetic signature enables scientists to see which part of the body is the cancer site. It would alleviate the necessity for a whole range of tests. The report concluded that it 'is still in development and a trial is being planned'. Soon, I hope. Soon.

I can sense that there is a powerful drug active in my system. I now have the occasional cramp. I have never been bothered with cramp in all my life. The arthritis in my knees is making me age as I walk with it. But really all of this is minor if the final result means a longer life. Life is so good and even though I know that one day it will end I want to do all I can to help my physical frame.

I know what all this is doing to my husband and I would have given anything to have spared him all this. We have been lovers, partners, mates for all of our fifty years together. In retirement we have written books together, interviewed people together, argued together, wrestled with ideas. Ours has been a fortunate life and we have talked very little to other people about the painful times unless we could help someone in the telling. I realise all too late that if you live hopefully people think, as one friend said after reading Ian's autobiography, 'that the sun had always shone on both of you'.

But such deep intimacy has its cost when one or the other partner becomes ill. At times Ian is unable to stop himself from saying things like 'We have had such a wonderful life, darling' and I hear it as if our life together is ending and I don't want to hear that. Not yet.

I am not in denial. How can I be when every morning I come out of the bathroom and am confronted with my prosthesis bras? The prosthesis still seems very heavy as I put it on and I can't believe my other breast weighs the same. Once I have it on there is no problem with the weight. But certainly denial is not a possibility.

7

We have had our two Hobart grandchildren with us. They arrived at Melbourne airport from Paris on Saturday afternoon. It was a good arrival time and before long they were through Customs and into the car.

Our grandson, the eldest of our seven grandchildren and now aged nineteen, was sporting a pair of quite extraordinary shoes in bright orange and blue which gave him, already a tall 185 centimetres, an extra four. Our grandson had negotiated his trip to London and back and managed to find his way around London. He had spent ten days there and the shoes were his treat to himself. I think to myself if you can't wear outrageous shoes at nineteen you probably never can. The Customs people in Vienna had put the shoes separately through their X-ray machine. I was not surprised.

Our granddaughter, soon to be fourteen, arrived with the bear she had taken all the way to Paris and back. They both seemed glad to be on terra firma after their long return flight but were uncomplaining. Their father and his fiancée are living in France for six months and had rented a very small Paris apartment for four weeks to show them the sights. My granddaughter described to us in graphic detail the minute bathroom that had a bath but where they could not shower because the ceiling was too low for them to stand up. The granddaughter is a born actress and we could see it all as she described sleeping on the sofa with her feet dangling over the edge. I couldn't help wondering whether, while away, my own son had thought about his time in Europe in 1977 when apart from the occasional postcard we had to push all our fears for his safety from our minds for six weeks. If only there had been mobile phones then.

This son is a born educator and made sure that the children saw all the tourist places, the Louvre, the Musée d'Orsay, the Pompidou Centre, the Tuileries, the Place des Vosges, The Luxembourg Gardens, Versailles on a hot day with all the fountains playing, Monet's garden at Giverny, markets, shops, all that a young teenager could enjoy. On her last day our son had asked his daughter if there was anything she especially wanted to do that she had not done. She had loved the area around Montmartre, the top of the Eiffel Tower at night, but she hadn't eaten snails. As a treat, the two of them went to a little bistro so that she could savour les escargots.

As they told of their escapades my mind kept running back to 1969 when as a family we had travelled through Europe in summer with a campervan and a tent. I was not a camper but Ian had taken the boys on camping trips and loved it and in any case we couldn't afford more luxurious accommodation. Jane and I were to sleep in the van and the boys and their father in the tent. Our second camping site wasn't far from the Bois de Boulogne and on this particular day we had taken the Metro into central Paris. We had left our sleeping bags in the tent with the flap opened just a few inches to let in some air. While we were away, the heavens opened and we returned to find our sleeping bags floating inside the tent. It was quite the worst night of our European holiday but I found myself thinking that any apartment, however small, would have been preferable to the hard floor of the tent or the uncomfortable division in the seats of the van where we slept.

Before we went camping I had gone to Marks and Spencers and bought tins of food and packets of instant potatoes. I thought that since the cooking in the van was restricted to two jets, speed of meal preparation would help. Most of the meals we enjoyed but there was one thing the children refused – Deb potatoes. There were still a dozen packets in the cupboard when we returned to London. I recall the goat's cheese we had bought at a local market in France which eventually filled the campervan with its powerful aroma and in exasperation our elder son had thrown it out the window.

All parents are different. Ian and I are both teachers, I thought, and although we weren't aware of it we were always showing and explaining, finding new things to delight and interest the children. Now they are in their forties they do the same thing to their offspring. So our son had made sure that the children were exposed to a wide variety of experiences knowing that some of them would only be appreciated five or ten years on.

In 1969 our camping journey had taken in France, Switzerland, Austria, Italy, Yugoslavia and Belgium, and it was not without its hazardous moments. We had spent time driving through the three Swiss passes, Susten, Grimsel and Furka, and had negotiated the steep downward slopes and onto the flat roadway. Fine rain began to fall and I suggested that we should stop and put our cases that were on top of the van inside it. As Ian put his foot to the floor, he realised that the brakes no longer worked. What if this had happened a few minutes earlier? We stayed at Andermatt until the brakes were repaired but it gave us time to take the cablecar up to the peaks, where the mountains seemed to go on forever into the distance. After lunch one afternoon we saw in the window of a shop a zither. It was old and the timber surrounding the strings was beautifully decorated with birds and flowers. It made a charming sound when the strings were plucked and in an impetuous moment we decided to buy it. It has gone down to the next generation.

I was always anxious about my mother's health during the sabbatical. My three brothers were all living in Melbourne, but I was the only girl and especially close to my mother and had hated leaving her in so much pain.

As we were driving up the Brenner Pass past the town of Fortezza there was the sound of an approaching police siren, a sound I thought peculiar to the Italian police. At first we thought they were after the car in front of us, but no, it was our van they were about to pull over. Fear gripped me. Something must have happened to my mother. We had very little Italian and could do nothing else but hand over our precious passports and follow the police back down the hill to the station. We waited and waited while long telephone conversations took place. We understood very little of what was being said and felt utterly powerless. Finally with more gestures and indecipherable words we were handed back our passports and dismissed. A mistaken number plate! We never did find out the whole story and we were now three hours behind schedule for our next camping place.

Some days were spent at a youth conference at Ruschlikon on Lake Zurich. Oh the bliss of a proper bed! Our Swiss hosts were very kind and on the evening of the Swiss National Day we all went by bus to a festival near the shore of Lake Lucerne. There were alpine horn quartets, yodelling, singing, dancing, and an extraordinary display of fireworks as a finale. In the middle of it all, our second son disappeared. He was the dreamer and inclined to wander off. This wasn't like a child lost in a store, this was someone lost with insufficient French or German to explain to anyone who he was. The whole party went off searching for him and eventually found him. He was quite unperturbed. I felt as if I had aged ten years.

In the 1960s, travel in Yugoslavia was limited and when we were eventually cleared to cross the border we encountered villages where little had changed over the centuries it seemed, and despite the beauty of the old town of Ljubljana the areas outside of it had the drab appearance of a communist regime. We purchased a small brass pepper grinder and a wooden flute-like instrument, beautifully carved, that made a marvellous sound.

In Austria we had spent several days with the family we had known since 1956. The children were of similar age and language didn't seem to be a barrier. They played cards, went swimming, went for walks and had a great time.

Now our son has done the same thing for his children, at some sacrifice but with enormous pleasure. We pass on these ways of parenting, never thinking of it going on from generation to generation. The first time I held the first of our grandchildren, I had the strangest feeling. I thought I could now understand the words 'from generation to generation'. Here was a new generation inheriting not only the family name but a whole genetic strain. Tully had grown up to look like his father, his grandfather and especially his great-grandfather. They had many of the same mannerisms, the same deep brown eyes. I loved watching my grandson talk to his grandfather. They seemed to be on the same wavelength.

I am not a shopper, really. That is not to say that I don't like beautiful things but I obey the dictum of (was it Miss Buss or Miss Beale?) to only ever buy something if it is necessary or very beautiful, and I have to confess that sometimes the beautiful had taken precedence over the necessary. Friends just assumed that I didn't want this or that practical item but often, especially in the first twenty years of our marriage it had been a deliberate choice. The beautiful picture, lamp or piece of furniture gave me and Ian so much pleasure. There is a lot of what is called 'stuff' in shops these days and most of it has little appeal for me. This is a time of getting rid of things rather than acquiring them.

I do, however, need to understand this young granddaughter who adores shopping, loves 'stuff' and can think of nothing better than an afternoon looking at clothes in frock shops. While I was in hospital I was given a beautiful hand cream that I would never have bought myself. It came from Buderim in Queensland and had the most delightful scent. I mentioned to my grandson that I had been unable to find it in the shops and he checked it up on the Net and told me where I could buy another tube. Why not go shopping with my granddaughter?

How do you not indulge a young teenager you only see once or twice a year most years? Spoiling was what grandparents were for, surely. I remembered envying friends who had grandparents, aunts and uncles when I was growing up. All I had was a great-aunt and an aunt. Not much, really, although my aunt had lived with us until she married a widower, and had been very kind to me..

It was June sale time. Lily has dark hair, brown eyes and olive skin tanned after a month of summer weather. Everything she tried on looked attractive on her. After much trying on and much walking up and down, we bought a deep pink blouse ('They're wearing deep pink in Paris, Grandma'), a light pink zippered jumper that would be warm in a Hobart winter and a long-sleeved top. I knew that I was enjoying it all as much as my granddaughter. Ian, generous as ever, just smiled at the female world he was observing. He doesn't understand shopping at all and a book or a CD gives him enormous pleasure these days.

My grazier son has had so much rain overnight after the long drought that he can't even take a horse out to the paddocks to feed the ewes and their new lambs. But rain. Such a relief. But there was sad news as well. My god-daughter's father had died. We had known the family since they had all lived in Adelaide, but when they moved to Perth after five years in India we saw very little of them. The same day I had news of a friend from my schooldays who was dying of cancer. I had spoken to her only a couple of months ago when she was fit and well. We had talked about renovating gardens, for not only was my friend a marvellous gardener, she was a superb potter. I had bought many pieces of hers over the years, not always for myself but as birthday gifts and wedding presents. I was always surprised that the glazes were changing, the style was changing and she had a distinctive 'voice' as a potter, the sort of 'voice' you know makes all the difference between competency and original ideas. She was always unassuming, but there was a sureness in all her creative work, whether cooking or gardening, felt-work or pottery. We had sat in the same row of the assembly hall all our secondary schooldays and I wanted to visit her but felt that it might be an intrusion and a letter could be better. We were not intimates, and I think there is nothing worse than the way people come into situations in a voyeuristic way. I thought I would think things through in the garden. Time in the garden always seemed to put everything in the right perspective. It takes me into a larger world somehow.

I am less fearful of scratches and thorns these days. In the early weeks after surgery I was very protective of my arm when gardening, but I have greater confidence at this stage of my recovery.

Ian has a large bag full of gardening and painting clothes. It amuses me whenever I look at it because the painting we do these days is minimal, but the gardening and painting clothes are on their way to a rag collection as their next stop. Ian pulled out a gardening jumper, a Herdwick jumper bought in the Lake District in 1977. I was surprised it was still free of moth holes, but thought that the tough Herdwick wool was too tough for moths. It was ideal for a day of sun but cold winds.

We had both a spring and an autumn holiday in the Lake District in 1977 staying with friends we had met in 1969 on our way home from a sabbatical year. On board ship were a host of children migrating to Australia with their parents and, tuning in to the anxiety of their parents, the children spent much of their time running madly around the decks. There were quite a number of returning schoolteachers sitting and observing their behaviour, all reacting in different ways, but certainly reacting. We talked to one another about it and before long we had decided to band together and offer a couple of hours teaching each morning in whatever subject we were competent in. After discussions with the purser, a notice about the school came out in the daily bulletin, one of the lounge areas was set aside and most of the secondary school children attended each morning. It gave their parents some breathing space and eased the apprehension of the students.

It was here at the 'school' that Ian, teaching English, met Gordon, teaching mathematics. Gordon and his wife, June, were on their way to visit June's sister in Melbourne and we spent quite some time listening with fascination to Gordon's stories of his time with the Indian railways and later of the home he and June set up in the Lake District for children whose parents were in the Colonial Service. Their own children were all grown up and married with children but they had a natural affinity with the young. They made Ian promise that on our next leave we would visit them in the Lake District. We did and in the spring Gordon suggested that we might like to have the use of their son's cottage at Near Sawrey in the autumn. The cottage was just down the hill from Beatrix Potter's house, now owned by the National Trust. She had been extraordinarily generous and had bought up large areas of land and offered them to the Trust to maintain the great beauty of the place she had loved. There is a soft autumn light that combines with misty mornings to give almost an air of unreality about the place. This coupled with the greenest of green fields, church bells ringing and the bleating of Herdwick lambs almost at our back door, all this must have made it a perfect setting for her imaginative stories of Peter Rabbit and his friends.

Ian has always been fascinated by the Victorians and only this morning told me that Beatrix Potter's father was a capable photographer and a friend of the artist Millais. He had photographed Millais' grandson in order to assist the artist in the famous painting that advertised Pears' soap and became known throughout the world as Bubbles. What many people never knew was that the curly-headed angelic boy in the painting became the distinguished admiral in the Second World War, Admiral Sir William James.

In places such as Lake Windermere the Victorians had built great houses and set them in spacious grounds far from the belching chimneys where they had made their fortunes. Tourists come in their thousands and many are expert climbers. The Hansen family attempted two steep climbs but were often passed by hearty middle-aged fell walkers. It was always worth the effort, especially the views from Striding Edge with the icy winds blowing, but we were somewhat aghast some weeks later to read in the newspaper that someone had fallen to his death while up on the Edge. It was fascinating at the top of the climb to watch birds of prey and ravens taking advantage of the swooping currents of air, tiny finches and lower down the slope sheep jumping gaily in the autumn-coloured bracken.

It was at Grasmere at the end of our holiday that we bought Ian and David their Herdwick jumpers. Clothes, if kept long enough, may provide a rich harvest of memory.

While we were in this tamed countryside I wondered how early settlers must have felt when confronted with the vast Riverina plains or any of Australia's inland's vast spaces.

We loved travelling and are incurable romantics. Ian had been invited to lecture in Australian Literature at the University of Venice during their winter term. While there we had taken the opportunity to spend New Year in Siena. I had remembered George Steiner saying to us at lunch that 'God is in Siena, but He is not in Florence.' We would see for ourselves.

Siena at the time was never crowded for the Christmas–New Year period and from Australia the only place we could book into was a converted palazzo whose prices were exorbitant, but I thought that after an overnight stay there we would be able to find somewhere less expensive. It was to be our one extravagance. The rooms, left in their original style, were magnificent with enormous fireplaces, beautiful tables and chairs, photos taken last century of the Gori Marciano household and old portraits of noblemen adorning the walls. Because there is a demand for luxury in a particular modern style, the bedroom's en suite had been modernised and there was glass and chrome everywhere. I suppose it is all a matter of personal taste, and the large bath and abundant hot water I enjoyed, but it all seemed too abrasive for its setting in the gentle countryside. The next morning we went down into the old city and found a room in the heart of Siena only a minute from the Campo.

First-time visits to places make an impact that is never possible on a second visit. In some ways television has dulled the moment of arrival somewhat. We know what sunset looks like from the cliffs at Santorini, the beauty of the Place de la Concorde, arriving and seeing as you walk out of the station the marvellous Grand Canal in Venice. Perhaps, I thought, this is why there is the great search always for the new and exotic place not yet found by hordes of tourists and photographed to death.

Siena is built on three hills and the streets and alleyways in its heart all lead down to the main Campo or square known for its famous horse race, the Palio. It is a glorious design, rather like an opened fan, and around the fountain of Della Quercia hosts of pigeons gathered.

At the time, our grandchildren were small and we had quite a collection of picture books and story books for them. Why not a story about a little pigeon in the Piazza del Campo? And so *Leonardo, the Pigeon of Siena* was born. It had a long gestation period waiting for the right illustrator but eventually it came to birth with just the right photographs and drawings to match the gentle tale of two pigeons who fall in love and make their home in the Mangia Tower. Ian's original story was much longer and with greater detail but the love story of Leonardo and Columba and the drawings of the city and the Tuscan countryside has appealed to readers over a long period and is still borrowed by children from libraries. It came out in 1998 with a dedication to our seven grandchildren, Angus, Annie, Douglas, Erica, Lily, Sam and Tully, who loved seeing their names in print.

Everyone who visits Siena has their own particular delights from the city. They have been in the crowds in the square for the Palio or have eaten its famous panforte but I remember it for its illuminated manuscripts in the library of the Duomo, the superb Pinturicchio paintings and murals, the exquisite mauve to blue of the clear night skies and the generous hospitality offered us in a small restaurant that faced out onto the main square. Here we dined most evenings, not just for the view, but for the grace and charm of waiters who served *vitello a la Sienese*, *tortellini alla panna*, veal marsala, ravioli, and tartufo and gelati – all dishes that can be eaten here at home in Australia but which in such a place and served with such grace and charm were rare treats.

8

This afternoon, with snow falling on the ranges and a maximum temperature forecast of thirteen degrees, we set off for Tullamarine to collect two suitcases sent from southern France by our son and his partner. They still have three months overseas and thought it best to lighten their travelling load.

I thought about our travelling. I had never travelled lightly, always anticipating a lack of drying facilities in a hotel or a sudden change in the weather. I know of friends who have their packing for work or holidays down to a fine art. Not for them the weight of a heavy case to be carried up endless station steps and stairs. The main problem for us was that our travelling had nearly always been associated with work and so more formal wear was necessary.

I laughed to myself as I remembered travelling home from Britain in 1970. All the bits and pieces taken on board the boat train to Southampton. Amongst our hand items were five sleeping bags, a zither, a clavichord, a painting and a large piece of sculpture. Our kind and generous English friends who had come to farewell us couldn't believe their eyes. But we were, after all, Orstralians!

The painting, a portrait of Monsignor Lapotte by Edwin Long (1829–1891), we had bought in a strange picture framer's off the Portobello Road market. We suspected that it was a sketch for a larger portrait and at the time it had a hole in the lower centre. Some years later when we could afford it we had it restored at the National Gallery of Victoria by Harley Griffiths and the priest's interesting face sits above the dining room fireplace. He seems almost part of the family! In his day Edwin Long lived close to the Brompton Oratory (where

Monsignor Lapotte was in residence?) and had earned the largest sum of any living artist for his grand paintings of biblical scenes, such as *The Babylonian Marriage Market*, *The Raising of Jairus' Daughter* and *The Flight into Egypt*. There are several of his canvases in the stacks of the NGV in Melbourne. I don't care for them at all but there is no doubting his skill as an artist. The sculpture, bought at this same fascinating framer's, was of a bear or perhaps a stoat. Nobody was prepared to hazard a guess. It has stood on a display cylinder in our hall for over thirty years and it is rare for a visitor not to touch it. It invites touching in the way a Henry Moore does. I often play the clavichord but its gentle sound demands recorders, flutes or lutes to accompany it.

It set me thinking about the baggage we carry with us, baggage from the past, baggage of the present and baggage of the future. Baggage from the past that we need to let go of if only because it is past: guilt, regrets, anger, hurt, fear. Baggage that prevents us enjoying the present moment because often our minds are full of unnecessary concerns, baggage of the future that spoils enjoying the present and the baggage of family relationships that weigh heavily because we want life for our family to be better than it is and often we ourselves can do nothing about family, but the baggage stays with us when we should let it go.

Only the other evening Ian and I had watched a program on the mountain climber Brigitte Muir who was determined to climb the highest peak on seven continents. In the interview she said an interesting thing: 'It is a lot harder to make something of your life at home. It is more difficult than climbing mountains.' But she went on to say that she finds inspiration in people now, not landscapes. Fear, she said, is always about the unknown and she had not been afraid when climbing because she knew about mountains.

I went to bed that night thinking about Brigitte's statement that it is all about challenging yourself. I'm not a Brigitte Muir but I think that I can tolerate a fair amount of discomfort. I have been on the new drug, Arimidex, for four weeks now. It may be a better drug than Tamoxifen but it isn't for everyone and for the moment it makes me lethargic and takes away my appetite. Cooking meals is no longer a pleasure and there are times in the day when I am reminded of my pregnancies and the nausea I felt then. But 'everything passes' and perhaps I will feel better when my system becomes accustomed to it.

It is the spring equinox today and the mere fact that we are moving into longer days is enough to make me enjoy the cosiness of the study in winter and the pleasure of reading in a warm, snug bed at the end of the day. Ian and I will go on reading all night if our novel or biography has caught our imagination. Usually we set a time now, and whatever the stage we are at when that time arrives we stop. I love the quiet, the stillness, the lack of traffic on midwinter nights. Now that our son has had follow-up rain I can enjoy the winter sunshine. Because of the long autumn the roses are still blooming and the pruning must wait for another couple of weeks.

It is interesting the way in which people prune roses. My husband is gentle and prunes patiently. It is as if he doesn't want to hurt the rose bush. I am much faster, more ruthless, less patient. I know what to make of that!

My father gave me a daphne bush some years before he died and I have nurtured it. Today it is coming into bloom and the jasmine is running along the fence at a great rate and its flowers are beginning to appear. I am not sure which is my favourite scent, but I think it is jasmine. Flower-arranging is always a pleasure and the bay tree's glossy leaves make a wonderful backdrop for whatever flowers I can find in the garden. This morning I notice that there are at least five small bay trees appearing nearby and I decide to pot them up for friends.

9

Much has been written about friends and friendship and it seems that most of us have people that come in and out of our lives. Acquaintances. Then there are friends. People we are always pleased to see, whom we keep in touch with but not always as regularly as we should, and then there are intimate friends. These are fewer in number, but we trust them implicitly. They know us, we know them and at different times we have both revealed our deepest hopes, fears, concerns to. When you have moved from place to place, written histories, you have the privilege of meeting dozens and dozens of people in the course of your writing. Teaching, whether at school or university, as in Ian's case, brings more people into your circle.

Only this morning we had a telephone call from a former student of Ian's. He had been one member of a class of very bright students he had taught during his first years of teaching at Adelaide Boys' High School in the 1950s. The student had entered the South Australian parliament, eventually becoming deputy premier of the state. He was visiting Melbourne and had looked Ian up in the telephone book. He spoke of the influence Ian had been on him as a student and was ringing to acknowledge this. It was a nice gesture and very affirming. It happens more regularly to Ian than he can sometimes believe. It is probably true of all teachers. We leave some sort of impression on our students. We hope they remember us with affection.

But these are acquaintances. Friends, however, can mean a lot to us when we are diagnosed with cancer. It is as if our antennae are up high all the time. If a friend says, 'You're looking well', we take heart because the progress of this strange disease cannot be plotted on a graph, it isn't like a broken arm or leg that can be X-rayed to see if the bones have knitted.

At this stage, seven months since surgery, there is no way of knowing how well things are going. A friend can inadvertently turn a good day into a bad one. They don't mean to reduce your buoyancy but 'After you left we were talking about you and thought you looked pale. Are you all right?' Terrific. Who wants friends? I'm sure they mean well, but empathy isn't something a lot of people do very well. On the other hand, real intimates can say the same thing but they know the moment and the way to phrase their concern. We're so fragile just under the surface. One of my sons tells me that the problem is my voice. It is always so bright. It isn't something new. It is just my voice inherited from a Scots mother and a Welsh father. But it is times like this when my husband who is lover, friend and companion means everything. And for that I can scarcely find words.

10

It is my Lutheran friend Trudi's birthday today. She will be eighty-seven. I met her about twelve years ago when Ian and I were invited to write the centenary history of the Lutheran school, Immanuel College, in Adelaide. So much of South Australia's history is tied up with English and German settlement and since Ian was born there and received all of his secondary education and his tertiary education there he was already familiar with the Lutheran presence. He had been taught by people with names like Pfitzner, Twartz and Schultz.

By the time we were offered this history, we had co-authored three books on commission and we knew something of what would be involved: interviewing old scholars, present students and staff, researching archives and so on. We knew too that it would mean numerous trips to and from Adelaide, but we also knew that the Lutheran Archives were some of the finest archives in the country and kept up to date by meticulous volunteers. Of course we knew schools, but we knew that this would be different. Men and women who believed passionately in education had set up a school in the broad-acre farming hamlet of Point Pass in the mid-north of the state.

Colin Thiele, the author, wrote so vividly of his childhood in that area in a German Lutheran household. Life was not easy for these pioneers. 'Good roads were rare: rutted tracks made travel time-consuming. The great clumsy German wagons jolted and bucked: the dour drivers in the intense summer heat sat under gum tree boughs lashed to the plank-seat for shade. Light buggies, for all the careful driving in the world, split spokes and broke axles. And life was hard for women. There were no stoves and they had to cook in cast iron camp ovens over a fire in the small kitchen which was detached from the living quarters of the house. They baked their own bread, carried water in kerosene cans balanced across a yoke, tended the garden with its vegetables, bought calico and linen by the yard and sat up late at night by candlelight sewing shirts, trousers, underwear and pillowslips. The children had little fun at home and played few games because they had to fill the woodbox, gather eggs, bring in cows and even the girls were expected to plough with a team of four bullocks,' or so we wrote together. Things were not much better when Leidig, the first headmaster, and his wife, newly arrived from Germany, came to the manse that would be eventually both school and home.

Adjacent to the church was the cemetery and I remembered how on our first visit north to the old school Ian and I had stood there reading the names and ages of all the young children who had died as a result of childhood illnesses... It wasn't just the tyranny of distance that the headmaster had to cope with, but droughts and the subsequent difficulty of finding school fees meant that payments often had to be paid in kind with bags of wheat or bales of hay.

But there had been something remarkable about the persistent and persisting life of this school. It had begun with two part-time teachers and two students. Martin Luther had talked about the God 'who can change the impossible into the possible and nothing into something'. The South Australian Lutherans believed in these possibilities. Throughout its now more than one hundred years it has been a welcoming community and in 1970 a Greek girl could say of the school,

> I spent the greatest years of my life at Immanuel. Immanuel was the kind of place where if you took the time to listen you could actually hear the future.

My friend Trudi had attended the school and regretted that fact that like so many girls at that time she had been unable to continue with the education that she had so enjoyed at the school when it was in its North Adelaide premises. What it had given her was the one thing

I hope all schools give their students: a desire for life-long learning and a lively curiosity about the world and everything in it.

I think that of all the histories and biographies we have written I am proudest of *With Wings*. It was giving back to a remarkable people their story. I looked again at the newspaper cutting with its review of the book. The reviewer had described the book as 'a robust history for a robust people…a story of a people, not just a school. Their hard life in South Australia is revealed with such realism we can almost hear the creaking windmills and the voices of children in class.' Ian and I couldn't have been more pleased.

It was a rare privilege to interview old scholars who told stories of day staff and boarding staff, of their hard work and sacrifice to give them a good education; they told of their treatment in two world wars when men were interned, when the names of streets and towns were changed and even the names of roses in the Botanical Gardens altered. They told all this without a trace of bitterness. That was just how it had been.

The settlers in the 1830s from Prussia were fleeing religious persecution but when they settled here they were, above all, South Australians. They were not transplanted Englishmen who in many instances viewed this land as a kind of second best. This was to be the land of their children and their children's children and they wanted the best for it. They considered education to be not just the right of every citizen but a necessity for the well-being of their adopted land. In their first thirty-five years in their new land they had established seventy Lutheran schools throughout the state. Such was the priority they gave to education.

I look at the photo of the young headmaster and his wife newly arrived from Germany. Both in their early twenties and so far from the land of their birth. Could we still strive to overcome difficulties in the way in which they had, I wonder.

Ian and I had been working on the final chapter of the book and wanted to be able to tie the present in with the past. It would not be easy to travel into East Germany but we wondered whether the landscape would reveal a sense of place: the old church, the fields, the river where the emigrants took the barges downstream to Hamburg. It would make a good epilogue. When we returned home we wrote our epilogue. There were parts of it that convinced us that the journey had been worthwhile. We had written in one part,

> On back roads and through village after village we begin to feel the landscape, the ploughed fields, a farmer sowing seed by hand, the woods of pine and birch and it seems that not a great deal has changed. We travel to Erfurt where a young Martin Luther came to study in 1501. We pass the house where the student Martin lodged, the Augustinian monastery where he trained to be a monk. We take the train to Eisenach and hurry by taxi up to the Wartburg, the ancient fortress where Martin Luther was hidden by Frederick the Wise. We marvel at the hard-working Luther who translated the New Testament into German in eleven weeks. Such industry shames us.

It is spring and there is snow, driving rain and biting winds while we are in the Wartburg castle but we know that it was also spring when this little group of people took the momentous journey on the Prince George to Australia. In the woods below the Wartburg were white anemones bursting from the snow-burnt ground, symbols of the kind of hope and courage they wanted to pass on to the next generation of Lutherans.

How did all this joint writing come about? I had been trained as a research librarian, Ian was a Reader in Education at Melbourne University. Both of us have always been interested in history but had no formal education as historians although Ian had written the centenary history of Camberwell Grammar and that had been very well received. Not long before Ian's retirement from the university he was invited to write the history of the Headmistresses' Association. The headmasters and headmistresses had decided to form one association. Part of the reason for this was that some of the leading boys' schools were becoming co-educational and so having separate conferences was obviously not the way forward. The former headmaster of Trinity Grammar School in Sydney had already written a very elegant history with the title *Our Proper Concerns*, about boys schools' headmasters, and it seemed only right that the women should be celebrated in a similar fashion. Would Ian be able to do it? I had recently retired from teaching and Ian suggested that if they were prepared to have us as joint authors we would be happy to do it. My headmistress at PLC had been one of the instigators of the association and I felt that like so many of these women my Miss Neilson had not received the recognition due to her.

Fortunately there were minutes of all their meetings and it wasn't difficult to enter into the changing world of the headmistresses. I thought of the schools I knew well these days. There were still single-sex girls schools but quite a number of single-sex boys schools had adopted co-education, not just as an educational philosophy but more often to soften the macho style of their boys or to suit the desires of the parents for co-education, or to make their schools economically more viable. It was Australia's bicentenary year and people were constantly reviewing the past with fresh eyes, seeking to understand from where the nation had evolved. The book was to be an account of these headmistresses in conference together, the issues they discussed, what they hoped for young women in the future.

It is easy to forget how far women have come since the late 1820s, when for the first time women were able to attend lectures at the University of London. Nevertheless, there was a girls' school in Launceston in 1845 and one in Perth in 1846. The first gathering of the Victorian headmistresses had taken place in Melbourne in 1905. These women were passionate about the education of girls; they had style and it was often a forceful style necessary when coping with council members. It was in the 1980s that the word 'calling' was replaced with the word 'career' and the new career headmistresses were often married, had reared their children through adolescence, had often been forced to make compromises in their marital and domestic arrangements. They were tough. They needed to be.

Hyland House were helpful publishers but there was a delay in delivery from the printers so we had loaded the boot of our rather old Peugeot with sufficient copies for the launch at the conference to be held at Shore in Sydney. We had friends in Canberra who had invited us to stay en route to Sydney but at Narooma we had trouble with the car's engine. It was able to be repaired temporarily but we limped into Canberra. Our generous friends offered us the use of their second car to make the journey to Sydney and we left the Peugeot in Canberra.

The book was duly launched at the conference. I had the feeling that the men weren't too sure about this joint authorship. Had Ian sold out to them by co-authoring this history? Even some of the women were a little apologetic about *Feminine Singular*. I had always believed in the book, not because of my writing but because of what the minutes of the Association of Australian Headmistresses revealed of these remarkable women and the contribution they had made to succeeding generations of Australian women. They had given the girls confidence to pursue their dreams and many had gone on to prominent careers, not always acknowledging the debt they owed their schools.

Australians are not too sure about their independent school system. We know that there shouldn't be such a gap between many government schools and independent schools. There has to be a better way to go and that may mean greater sacrifices on the part of big schools in the funding of often massive structures for sport, drama and so on. In a recent book by George Steiner, *Lessons of the Masters*, he describes teaching as a privileged craft and the relationship between teacher and student as critical for any society. Like our now enormous houses that we build to seek status for ourselves, so with our schools. Parents should not be 'clients' or 'stakeholders', they should not be dictating to schools the nature of the education to be given to their offspring. Threats of legal action have brought fear into the hearts of many principals who need to have their confidence restored and be able to tell their boards, governing bodies or councils that as principal their central role is that of an educator and that is not the same as a CEO of a company. There is a need for the expertise of accountants, business men, and entrepreneurs, but they need to see their involvement as advisers rather than directors.

I thought of the years that had passed since I left teaching. I am tired of seeing uniforms change at regular intervals, of new signs at school gates, imposing buildings and showy advertisements.

Of all the reviews of *Feminine Singular*, I was most pleased with one by feminist Dale Spender, who described it as 'a well-written history, lively and analytical'.

While we were in Sydney I had used my research librarian skills and discovered that there was a Peugeot Car Club. I rang the number and a charming woman telephoned back the next day with the name of a Peugeot Car Club member in Canberra whom she was sure would be able to help us. When we returned to Canberra over a weekend the club member, a senior public servant and part-time rally driver, replaced parts and rebuilt the engine to fine working order, charging only for the spare parts.

So that was the beginning of our joint writing and from it all our other books followed.

11

Our grandson and his partner came for dinner tonight. They have never lived interstate before and are adjusting to so many changes in their lives. I want to nurture them in an unobtrusive way and thought that probably the best way was through food. I prepared a three-course dinner and roasted a chicken for them to take back to their communal house, where everyone seemed to eat nothing but tofu and lots of fruit and vegetables. All of it probably healthy enough but not ideal for a pair accustomed to a diet of red meat, chicken and fish.

Of course they were very polite at the dinner table and I told them that the food would only be wasted if they did not eat it, so they were able to eat large portions with ease. They are both tall and slim and there is little danger at the moment of them putting on too much weight.

As they sat together on the sofa I watched them, he with his arm gently around her shoulders, wanting to be protective of her. It crossed my mind that perhaps I wouldn't live to see them married, if in fact they did want marriage eventually. All I really wanted was to live long enough to be there when my grandson's sister completed her Year 12. She is currently in Year 8.

Daughter and granddaughters. How little I had understood about life until after my fifties. Two granddaughters and a grandson I have only seen twice in the last twelve years. Family relationships are a complete mystery to me. Until they had married, all my children were close and to watch them together gave me such pleasure. Now my daughter is locked into a relationship that isolates her from family and friends and although Ian and I have tried to mend fences the situation seems unlikely to change. While in hospital I had written to my daughter telling her to watch her breasts carefully, just in case there was a genetic link. Both my mother and grandmother had died young, so I couldn't be sure. For a time after sending the letter I had hoped that there might be a call from interstate or perhaps a card. But nothing. I wonder sometimes just how much grief any one person could take. The sight of the two young lovers sitting together on the sofa gave me enough happiness to bind up my wounds, if only for a time.

12

It isn't easy to remain optimistic day after day when the days are short. I don't mind the rainy days when I can tuck myself up in the study and write but most days there is just enough light rain to produce high humidity and my system doesn't care for it. It is necessary sometimes to go out and refresh yourself. One of my favourite times from our years at Haileybury College had been to drive around the bay. The seascape and the clouds were always a delight and never the same. It had such a variety of moods. Yesterday it was as still as a mill pond, the water was a milky shade and there was scarcely a breath of wind to move the almost becalmed yachts.

Last days of any art exhibition are often crowded. The Mornington Peninsula Art Gallery was showing Venezia Australis: Australian Artists in Venice 1900–2000. It had been curated and planned by the Castlemaine Art Gallery. In a stylish catalogue Peter Perry quoted Hans Heysen, one of the earliest Australian artists to visit Venice: 'Venice is a dream. It is too beautiful – all and more than I ever imagined.'

The Streetons were in Venice on their honeymoon and Arthur had painted while Nora read. Perhaps it was the honeymoon, or the city or the vitality of the inhabitants or the spring sunshine. Whatever the reason, three or four of the Streetons in the exhibition positively glowed on the walls. They seemed brighter and almost livelier than any other Australian painting I had seen.

In the entrance foyer there were a number of paintings of Albert Tucker's *Rock Pool, Blairgowrie* series. The sea is always difficult for artists to capture, but here Tucker had managed to produce scenes that were quintessentially Australian. The water seemed just right and there was a cheerfulness about them that was engaging. Why do galleries never reproduce as postcards the paintings you want as a reminder of your visit? I am sure there is a valid reason, but there were no Tucker postcards.

Venice in the winter of 1977 was our first visit. We had booked ahead two rooms in a small hotel on the Grand Canal just down from the Doges Palace. In the seventies and in winter Venice was not as it is today and I could remember standing at one end of St Mark's square when it was covered with a thick coating of snow. There was not a soul in sight and we could see a small dog's footprints as it had scurried across the empty ballroom-like space. It was magical.

Then with two teenagers we had rushed madly from place to place, church to church, gallery to gallery, in the few days we had before leaving for Paris and Cambridge. But in 1983 Ian was lecturing at Professor Hickey's invitation to Italian students studying Australian literature. This time our room looked over the Grand Canal with ever-changing light day and night. My favourite moments were when the lights came on all over the city and there seemed an intake of breath by its inhabitants. At breakfast we ate our rolls and coffee in a breakfast room where the linen was a delicate pink and where we could observe elegant Italian women alighting from their *vaporetto* on their way to work. Sunrise touched the water with a pink wintry glow.

I had kept a brief diary so I knew that on our first morning we had gone to the Rialto market and although it wasn't early there were still porters hauling boxes of squid, flounder, crabs, ling, sardines and eels, and wondrous stalls specialising in chicken, sausages and cheeses, not to mention all the fruit and vegetables. One cheese stall had what was described as a *torta formaggio*, a cheese torte. It appeared to be made of blue-vein cheese layered with other cream cheese and a swirl of cream on the top.

We had watched a pasta maker turning out vast amounts of pasta sheets. Now, of course, people often have machines in their homes and make their own ravioli, tortellini and so on, but I had never seen so much pasta being produced at close hand before.

Venice is a city of surprises. On our way back from the market we had opened a church door, walked inside and found a ceiling covered with paintings by Tiepolo and amongst them was a resurrection to take your breath away.

It is never easy to see everything in a city of so many treasures. We loved the mosaics in St Mark's, especially the Creation and Noah letting his bird out from the Ark. There is so much artistic extravagance everywhere. The light fitting in our room was Murano glass in the form of a cluster of daffodils and in the centre of each flower was a light bulb; it would have looked over the top anywhere else but in Venice it seemed just right.

The Riva degli Schiavoni, the thoroughfare beneath our window, was always crowded with families at weekends. We were never sure whether to watch from our windows or join the throng.

We were woken one morning by clanging bells from churches all over the city. Although no longer observed as a holiday, the bells rang for Epiphany.

The University of Venice is a converted palazzo and I was reminded of this when looking at one of the Streeton paintings taken from the top of Palazzo Foscari. Most people take romantic gondola rides in Venice. We had crossed the canal regularly in a *traghetto*, where the occupants stand as they are taken across the canal. It is necessary to concentrate to maintain your balance. One late afternoon purely by chance we had come upon a procession of gondolas and other small craft moving down the canal with bands and blazing torches that made ripples of golden light all the way along the canal.

It was all right to buy a roll or a pizza square for lunch but the evening meal at the hotel didn't fit our budget. I had seen what appeared to be a friendly family restaurant just around the corner from the hotel and we eventually became known as *gli Australiani*. One evening there was a group of Australian teachers eating there and we had a great time together. The restaurant served spaghetti, ravioli with clam sauce and beautiful fresh fish served in a variety of ways. For me it was always a pleasure at the end of the day to draw back the curtains in our room and observe the traffic on the canal, hear the mewing of the odd gull, delight in the pink lights along the pavement.

At High Mass at St Mark's on Sunday morning there were few people about. The sun shone through the windows on the golden mosaics, candles burned on the altar and incense rose as the bells clanged and the choir sang. These were both inner and outer moments for me. So very different from anything I had ever experienced before. So very different from any other worship experience. All so rich: the altar boys in their long black gowns, the celebrant in his red robe with white lace and an embroidered gold cope. The Bible readings were read beneath a gold-domed canopy and the choir's Sanctus was so very different from that in the Salzburg mass. Sunday afternoons were obviously for families and they were all out walking along the Riva with the children eating ice creams or carrying balloons or bags of goldfish.

One night the two of us dined with Professor Hickey. Good food, good conversation and it got late so we had a choice of hoping for the last *vaporetto* or walking back to our hotel. By now a thick mist had rolled in and you couldn't see your way ahead except for the lights. The bells were muffled, the fog horn sounded and our footsteps echoed as we walked down the narrow streets. A black cat ran across our path but everything else was so still. The gondolas moored in the side canals moved gently up and down as the water slapped against their sides.

For many years Ian had worn bow ties. I couldn't remember when he first wore them, but they had become part of his identity and he never wore anything else with his shirts. I loved window shopping in Venice and had found a little shop that made its own bow ties. At home hand-tied bow ties were expensive and there wasn't a great variety but here it was tie paradise. Before coming to Venice I had read in Jan Morris's book that clothes were important to the Venetians and that only the tourists looked scruffy – hence the bow ties.

Bernard Hickey had invited us to an evening at a salon where a film of Wagner in Venice was to be shown. We had walked through a pair of ordinary doors into an exotic room of chandeliers, and glittering women and obviously powerful men. Bernard Hickey was always giving us new experiences and he insisted that after the film we should go to Florians, the famous café frequented by Wagner. Bernard chose the drinks which were magnificent concoctions served in silver holders as extravagant as the music of Wagner we had been listening to earlier.

It would not be Carnivale for three weeks but I found a shop selling a wondrous array of exotic masks placed on models. One costume in green and gold was matched by an elaborate turban and a gold mask. Another outfit was in gold and silver with a ruffled collar that gave it the appearance of an Elizabethan courtier. By a side canal I discovered a mask maker and I walked in hesitatingly, for my Italian was far from perfect. However, I was able to negotiate the purchase of a beautiful sun mask that now hangs on our dining room wall as bright as the day I bought it from the charming young man.

The word 'ghetto' is thought to have originated from the site of an iron foundry and to get to it we had to take the *vaporetto* to San Marcuola and walk. The area is still predominantly Jewish. The lower windows were covered with grills and the craftsmen in the area were busy making Jewish plates, menorah and goblets in a place where still stands a sixteenth century synagogue. In 1943 and 1944 Jews were taken from here to concentration camps and Ian and I looked with sadness on a sculpture depicting firing squads and labour camps with barbed wire fencing at the top of the piece. A tablet nearby gave details of the events that had taken place. The faces we saw could have come from suburbs in Melbourne where Jews predominate. At the time the ghetto had not been just for Jews but for all foreigners and that had included the British ambassador.

After days of fog we decided to make a train journey to Padua to escape. Because of the fog the *vaporetti* were not running so we had quite a walk to the railway station. Venetians are very philosophical about the fogs that roll in frequently at this time of the year, but we found them claustrophobic.

Once out of the lagoon we discovered that it had snowed the previous night and our journey was a paradise of white willows, vineyards that appeared to be strung with long white cobwebs and tall grasses waving like giant white feathers. It seemed as if the snowfall had been followed by a frost that had sealed everything in this ravishing landscape. We had gone to Padua chiefly to see the Schrovegni Chapel decorated by Giotto. It is an intimate space full of frescoes of the life, death and resurrection of Christ and the whole back wall depicts the Day of Judgement.

Italian churches always have attractive nativity scenes for children to enjoy over the Christmas–New Year period, and in the church of St Anthony as well as a beautiful crucifix by Donatello and altar carvings there was a nativity scene to delight any child's heart. Everything seemed to move. There were oxen chewing their cud, shepherds bowing low at the crib, a mill wheel turning, a steaming cauldron on a fire inside a house, a boat sailing on distant waves, shepherds on a hillside warming themselves by a fire, sunrise and later sunset, and angels flying across the sky looking like every Italian angel ever painted.

Now most television viewers have seen travel programs depicting the first anatomy theatre for medical students in Padua. The first in the whole of Europe, it was built in 1594 and with its seven tiers there was standing room for three hundred students. The cadaver to be shown and dissected was brought up from a central well. The room where medical students still take their vivas has a single chair for the candidate and a semi-circle of seats for the examiners. This hall is sumptuous with coats of arms over the centuries, beautifully carved and gilded chairs which they may not notice during their ordeal.

By the time we returned to Venice, the fog had lifted and the *vaporetti* were running again.

Being in Venice, I thought, had been like attending a great feast. That wonderful memorial to preservation from the Great Plague is the seventeenth century basilica of S. Maria della Salute. It has Tintoretto's beautiful *Wedding at Cana*. Freshly cleaned, it has I think some of the loveliest faces of women in the whole history of art. Just around the corner from our hotel was the fifteenth century church of Saint Zaccaria with its *Virgin enthroned with the Saints* by Bellini. There was always music playing in the church and we frequently slipped inside to look at it on our way to somewhere else. On a foggy morning we had photographed what surely must be one of the world's finest equestrian statues, Verrochio's *Colleoni*, a mercenary who left money to have this statue erected upon his death.

It is small wonder that Venice attracts so many tourists; so many sights and sounds. Out shopping for lunch, I had seen a woman lowering a basket down on a rope from a top storey so that the postman could put her mail in it. Pigeons everywhere, not at all anxious to get out of the way as people passed. I had read somewhere that they were part of an ancient tradition where on a special day of the year the cities which were subject to Venice used to send the Doge a pair of pigeons. These were immediately set free over the Square of St Mark's. Protected and fed by the state, they come at the striking of the campanile at nine a.m. and two p.m. to be fed grain. It is no wonder they walk about so proudly. There were always housewives busy doing their shopping and fish stalls and greengrocers' stalls were scattered down alleyways.

On a Sunday of yet again thick fog, we took the train to Trento, a three-hour journey. Fishermen from the lagoon had put their nets out to dry in the mist but after half an hour we were in brilliant sunshine with blue sky and sun-capped mountains. The famous Council of Trent was held from 1545 to 1563 in the Duomo. The Chiesa di San Lorenzo, built in the twelfth century, had an interior rather like a stage setting with stone stairs leading up to the altar, and what was even more surprising were the enormous bowls of flowers decorating the church. Roses, nerines, lilac, irises and gerberas, they were extravagant and seemed to typify the generosity within the city. What is it that so quickly conveys the atmosphere of a place to a visitor? It wasn't the statue of Dante, who died there, or the frescoed buildings surrounding the square; rather it came from the people. In Trento everyone seemed charming; the girls that had served us coffee and torte, the young couple seated at a nearby table with a small baby, the little old lady who had sold us mandarins had all smiled warmly and were so welcoming. The sun was setting, there were pink and mauve clouds against the sky as we walked around the square with the floodlit fountain and floodlit square, and at six-thirty we boarded the train back to Venice.

Professor Hickey was always doing things on the spur of the moment. While Ian was lecturing to his students one afternoon he invited the two of us to a lecture followed by dinner with the speaker and his wife at the Hotel Londra where Tschaikovsky had written his 8th Symphony. We all drank champagne out of beautiful hand-blown glasses and the meal of pâté, pasta, veal and side dishes concluded with exquisite dolci made by the hotel's chef. By now it was eleven o'clock. It had been a full day and we were both ready for bed. But not Bernard. He thought it would be a good idea if the three of us went back to the apartment of one of the guests. Her flat was on the first floor of a converted theatre near the Rialto. The approach was similar to any other old Venetian palazzo but there was a beautiful entrance doorway, a marble foyer and stairs that were lit by lamps of the palest pink, green and mauve glass that threw their colours onto the marble. It was quite the grandest room I had ever entered, with paintings the size normally reserved for galleries, magnificent furniture, fine Persian rugs and everything in impeccable good taste. We sat and drank grappa until one a.m., when we felt it only proper to take our leave. As we walked back to the hotel I said to Ian, 'How are we ever going to settle back into normal life?' But I knew that a diet of cream puffs all the time was not for most people.

'Chiuso' on a sign outside a church, gallery or building was always an irritation to tourists who had only forty-eight hours to spend but Ian and I had been there for weeks and had never been able to get inside Vivaldi's church. However, we did see a great deal. Carpaccio was commissioned to decorate a chapel dedicated to Saint George, Saint Trifone and Saint Jerome, the three protectors of Dalmatia. The artist seemed to have enjoyed this commission. There was to my eyes so much amusement and keen observation in the work. The pictures all looked like something from a fairytale in the small space with its inlaid walls and carved pews. There was the familiar St George slaying the dragon and Saint Jerome and the lion, Saint Augustine's vision and many others.

We were enjoying a quiet lunch with Bernard when he asked me if I would be the hostess for an Australia Day function. He would be lecturing on Miles Franklin, and they would need champagne and about a hundred *dolci*. 'Just shop around, dear,' he said. How could I resist such a charming man? But one hundred *dolci*!

After Ian's time with his students we returned to the hotel on our usual *traghetto*. I was getting quite good at balancing standing up in one, and in any case there was a Tiepolo sky, so beautiful that nothing else seemed to matter.

We spent the following Saturday on Burano, the island of lacemakers, of multi-coloured houses with dark green shutters, of singing canaries and where fishermen sat in the winter sunshine mending their nets with as much skill as the women made their lace.

Torcello is so very different from Burano and the day we visited it the wind was blowing and the sky was overcast. It reminded me of the East Anglian fen country. There was a sense of desolation but also of past grandeur about the island. It had been great and it was from here that material had been taken for the building of Venice and the eleventh century cathedral still contains seventh century remains. At the time we were there the magnificent *Madonna with the Saints* was being repaired but the thirteenth century *Day of Judgement* glittered with some quite terrifying mosaics. A nearby museum had artefacts from Roman times. Today there are only a hundred inhabitants and it was hard to imagine that at one time it was home to twenty thousand. There were cats everywhere as we walked around, an odd rooster crowed, the bells of Burano floated across the water and it was a place where time seemed to stand still.

I had bought the wattle, the *dolci* and the champagne, going out in thick fog for my purchases. I had tied up the wattle with gold ribbon and had put all the sprays on the balcony with the bottles of champagne, away from the central heating of the hotel. Bernard gave a fine lecture and the celebration of Australia Day seemed to go off very well. Coming at the end of our time in Venice it seemed a fitting 'thank you' for all that the city had given us. The day we left the sun was shining as we travelled down the Grand Canal for one last time. I knew that the sights, smells, sounds and friends in Venice would always be like honey in my hive of memories.

13

I went with Ian to see my oncologist this morning and we had a long chat about Arimidex versus Tamoxifen and we both agreed that I should stay with Arimidex for the next two months. I still feel that Tamoxifen gives me a better quality of life. I have more energy when I am on it, but it seems only right to give the Arimidex time to settle into my system. I spoke to him about the constant enquiries about my health by well-meaning friends and he likened it to the way in which when a woman is pregnant everyone feels able to comment on her size, weight gain and so on and say how pregnancy had been for them. Very odd.

It was a bleak, grey winter morning and we all talked about the gloomy winter days in England and how quickly the days seemed to end and the long winter nights causing you to long for sunshine and blue skies. The oncologist is such an empathetic man and Ian is able to relate easily to him too. I suppose that because he is younger than my two sons he probably sees us as he would his own parents. Whatever the reason, it is always a positive experience to visit him and the sky seems brighter as we walk back to the car.

The next day we had friends for lunch and one had brought us a copy of *Uni News*. In it was an article urging women on HRT (hormone replacement therapy) to be extra vigilant about having their two-yearly mammogram. It appears that mammogram sensitivity is reduced in people taking HRT and higher breast density is associated with an increased risk of breast cancer. It said, 'Breast density indicated by the glandular tissue in the breast that appears white on a mammogram is higher in some women taking HRT which makes it more difficult to find breast cancer. Higher breast density is part of the reason why tumours are not detected in these women but we believe other factors also come into play.' So now I knew why it was that my cancer had not shown up clearly on the mammogram, I thought. Perhaps I was wrong but somehow it helped me to think that despite my best efforts it is always possible to miss it. An MRI plus the mammogram possibly would have made the difference. But who knows? To live is surely to live with risk.

That same week there was a report of work being done at the Walter and Eliza Hall by an old boy from my sons' school. He is working on 'the identification and characterisation of mammary stem cells... inspired by recent observations that cancers arise in organ-specific stem cells and retain stemcell-like properties that contribute to their malignant behaviours. If shown to be true, these observations have the potential to change the way cancer is treated.' So there was always new research going on. The sad news for me was that he is moving to the US next year, possibly because there are more research grants there.

14

I am pleased to have two postcards from our son in Paris. The London bombing caused much anxiety when I knew he would be in London for a wedding the next weekend.

Ian and I leave tomorrow for a week with our son in country New South Wales. He manages a property of fifty-two thousand acres and it is an eight-hour drive from Melbourne. Part of me would rather be at home with warmth, my writing and my books in winter, but I know how much our son is looking forward to our visit. We had planned a visit just before my cancer diagnosis and that seemed such a long time ago. He makes such a fuss whenever we visit and it brought to mind the journeys Queen Elizabeth I used to make to the stately homes of England. There certainly couldn't have been greater thoughtfulness or anticipation of a visit. I hope that the road into the property won't be like an ice rink. They have had seven inches of rain in four weeks after almost four drought years and it makes driving once off the bitumen a bit hazardous, not to mention the drive from the gravel road into the property. I knew that most of the dirt roads and part of the Cobb Highway had been closed due to rain.

As we left home I reflected on the number of times we had driven up to the Riverina in the past thirty-two years. The first was when our son had decided to leave the university and go jackerooing. It had been a very wet spring and our station wagon had slid off the slippery road into the table drain and a tractor was needed to get us out. We have travelled north many times since but I have never grown accustomed to the sliding and slithering on the red, saturated soil.

Small wonder people love the outback. Once we left Echuca,

the landscape was one of gorgeous tumbling white clouds above the horizon for a hundred and eighty degrees. The country had already greened and the air was crisp and clear, with the car's thermometer reading eleven degrees.

There is so much of our past in this journey north – births, a christening, a shattered relationship, different properties and now a new daughter-in-law-to-be and a university-aged grandson and another away at boarding school. We were staying overnight with our son's fiancée and I knew that it would be a strain. First visits are always like that. But I already love this widowed woman for the happiness she has brought to my son.

When we arrived there was a roaring fire downstairs and there were fresh flowers beside my bed. Our two grandsons came over before dinner. It was university and school vacation and it was an opportunity for us to see our grandson's car now fitted out with blue lights inside and the usual thumping sound system that young males delight in; the car was immaculate. His first semester at university had been a learning experience in so many ways. He was in shared student accommodation and had discovered how to make his allowance work by shopping well, learning the price of things and discovering quick ways of preparing meals and juggling study time with social time. Schools can never really prepare their students for this transition. Relationships can often take over the whole of a boy's life and before too long he is burning the midnight oil to make up for lost study time. There is no one there to prod him if he neglects his work. There is house cleaning, washing clothes and ironing all to be attended to.

They are such warm, affectionate grandsons and spending time with them gives me so much pleasure. Whenever I am with them my mind races back to when they were babies, then toddlers, walking with them along the airstrip of the property with a magnifying glass showing them ants and other tiny creatures. When they were older we played golf on their back lawn or they would take me to see the bike jumps they had made in a far paddock. It was hair-raising for a grandmother to watch the bike jumps but then I remember the risks my own sons had taken in their teenage years. It seems to be a necessary rite of passage for boys. The grandsons were always willing to help when they came out at weekends from boarding school. They would climb on the roof and clear the gutters, carry heavy garden pots for me or put down stepping stones made from the trunks of the old gum trees. They could do these things in half the time it would have taken me or Ian. I think that one of the chief roles of a grandparent is to affirm grandchildren, give them confidence in themselves.

As one of them talked about his university girlfriends, I wondered whether a society where marriages were arranged would not be better than some of the disastrous liaisons that occur when people are given free rein in their choice of partner. They are told so much about the necessity of good Year 12 results, of good study habits, but so little is ever said about the choice they will eventually make of a life partner. I have read somewhere recently that it will soon be quite common for people to have two and three marriages and I fear for some of the offspring who will have to cope with the results of these freedoms. Plenty of money and a high status career are fine, but a loving relationship doesn't always go with them.

Just after dinner tonight the heavy rain began again. The clothesline is full of washing and our son says that there hasn't really been any need for a clothesdryer until now but he thinks it may be a necessity if rain patterns return to normal. The sound of rain on the roof when we went to bed was such a treat, such a musical sound. We had arrived minus a hubcap and our son was quite sure that it must have been dislodged when we came off the bitumen. I hadn't heard or seen anything at the time but the gravel made so much noise and we were both concentrating on the enormous potholes full of water. Our son insisted on going back to the gravel road and, sure enough, the hubcap was exactly where he had predicted it would be.

The old homestead is beautiful and the main bedroom has two long windows that look from the bed out onto the front garden, with its tall palms and ancient jacaranda. The winter dawn chorus wasn't as loud as at other times of the year and I could only hear corellas and a lone crow. There was a large fireplace in the bedroom and in front of it our son had placed the tapestry screen worked by my mother many years ago. When she had come out from Scotland as a teenager with her grandmother, they had brought with them a piece of barghello tapestry that I had used to cover a bedroom stool. Peter was the only grandchild who had been old enough to know his grandmother well. He was the sentimental one of my three children and the only one interested in the firescreen.

What have I created that will be left behind when I am gone, I thought. People left finely knitted baby shawls that were passed on from children to grandchildren and even to great-grandchildren. They left exquisite embroidery, pottery and paintings. I have always been musical. Perhaps some will remember my playing, but flower arranging doesn't last longer than a few days and a finely prepared meal is soon demolished. My creativity is in my writing and I hope that the creative ideas I have given to family and friends will be my legacy.

I showered, had breakfast and walked outside. The washing was even wetter than when it was put on the line. But the Lachlan was rising fast and moving more quickly than yesterday. The ancient trunks of the river gums stood out against the lush green grass that seemed more like Spring green than midwinter green. Reading the local paper I had discovered that the new grass wouldn't provide sufficient nutrients for the sheep until three weeks after it first appeared. So it seemed that the end of the drought was even more complex than the city people understood. Hundreds of lambs had died when the rains came because their mothers, already weak from the drought, were deprived of their feed. Not even on horseback was it possible to get food to them, and the men couldn't bear to think of the sheep in those far paddocks that they had nurtured all through the years of drought.

The old homestead is full of character, with its flame mahogany furniture, its high varnished pine ceilings and its encircling veranda.

The guest wing is adjacent to the main home and always reminds me of something from the Raj. There is a sitting area, a long wide wire-screened walkway and bedrooms and bathroom.

Our son doesn't fit the image of a grazier that city people have. He writes, paints, and enjoys the environment he lives in. When he went there, he changed the furniture around, put paintings on the walls, polished the silver and made sure that it was somewhere where he could relax at the end of the day. Despite his heavy workload, Ian and I felt he managed his staff, the necessary bookwork, the care of his dogs and the holiday time with his sons remarkably well. The time since his divorce had not been easy and we will be glad when he has his new wife with him. His fiancée is travelling the three hours to be here for dinner and will stay for the weekend. Like all country women she handles distance with ease and never complains. My son is very fortunate.

The next day was one of blue skies at last and sunshine. We put out table and chairs on the front lawn and had champagne and a platter for lunch. The mulga parrots were everywhere and their blue and green feathers were gorgeous in the sunlight. We all went mushrooming that morning and found enough to make soup for the next day. There is such abundance. The orange, lemon and grapefruit trees are heavy with fruit and there are enough pumpkins in the store to last the year. The gardener keeps the herb garden alive and in the summer there will be grapes, figs and plums. Breakfast the next morning reminded me of formal English breakfasts with kidneys, bacon, mushrooms, eggs and freshly squeezed orange juice. The wind had sprung up and the ground was beginning to dry out but it was impossible to get to the far paddocks. I didn't fancy walking through the heavy mud. Some Italian boys had been given permission to go hunting wild pigs on the property but an old boar had defeated them, taking on all five of their dogs. A wild pig will devour a lamb a night but fortunately their numbers are down because of the drought. It hadn't been a good weekend for the boys; the river was too muddy for them even to get any fish.

The last time we were on the property the temperature had stayed in the forties for days on end and we only went outside when necessary or after the sun had set. The contrast with the weather now was extraordinary. This morning there was a hard frost, the third in a row, and we were coming up to full moon. I looked outside from the warmth of the bed and the sun was shining, but one step out of bed and I knew that it would be some time before there was any warmth from the sun. I settled back in bed with my book and enjoyed the luxury of a late start to the day.

One of the young staff has a litter of pups and wants to introduce them to the sheep. He takes them over to the yards. They are only twelve weeks old but already know what to do when put in with the sheep. I find this inbred, instinctive way of handling the sheep amazing. There is no fear in these tiny creatures; they know what they have to do.

Peter's fiancée has left for home. She is a delightful, vivacious girl with a friendly manner and to see her sitting with our son is to see two people very much in love. I thought of my sons' marriages with their first wives. They had come from very different backgrounds and had very little in common, really, but they had fallen in love and like all lovers believed that everything would work out. Both the boys and their wives had lived interstate so Ian and I hadn't seen a lot of them but I had tried to have good relations with them whenever they visited. Now the boys have new partners and I am much older and, I hope, a little wiser. If the women like me and we are able to relate well to each other, I will be pleased, but if not, then I can live with that. Ian and I have no need for anyone but each other now. I don't want to be self-centred or selfish but I am realistic enough to know that years don't stretch a long way into the distance. There is not a lot of time left to store honey in the hive and I am able to draw on all that has been put away over the years.

Ian and I could quite happily sit out on the lawn in the sun reading this morning and our son can't quite understand why I am not anxious to slide about in the ute to feed the calves. There was a time when I wanted to see everything on the property and explore every paddock. Not now. I am here with the dogs and am quite content. The busy city is so far distant that I can forget everything that waits for me there. Here there is just the sound of the odd fly buzzing around my head, the mournful cry of a crow, the sweet sound of the parrots and the chirp of the willy-wagtails. I wish I had been a twitcher, a bird-watcher, and could name the distant birds' songs. Suddenly there is the familiar laugh of the kookaburra, the first I have heard since we arrived.

There isn't a cloud in the sky today. The drenching rain that broke the drought seems to have gone, at least for a while, and everyone is enjoying the sun. It is easy for country people to see the big issues, the things that really matter, what it means to live well, when they are so far from the little things that intrude into life in a big city. There was a time when I would have found the distance, the stillness, the solitude a little threatening perhaps, but not now.

There is a crop duster flying low over a nearby property today. It is strange to hear the sound of an aeroplane. After sitting and writing in the sun, I went inside to begin preparing the evening meal, only to discover that since our morning's coffee there was no water coming out of the taps. There was always tank water in the refrigerator but after cooking the dishes would have to wait until someone returned from the paddocks to set the pump going. They are lamb-marking today. Part of yesterday was spent feeding out a liquid mixture of urea and molasses to the cows and young calves. One lot hadn't sampled it before and came up to the container with some hesitation. There were fewer mushrooms today. Perhaps we need to try another paddock.

Almost full moon and at night the paddocks are bathed in that mystical light stretching over the still countryside. Until the new moon there may not be any more rain but when we left this morning there was thick ice on the windscreen and the car's temperature gauge was flashing at -0 degrees for quite a few kilometres. It had been a sharp frost and it took a long time for the temperature in the car to climb.

Ian and I were both on the lookout for kangaroos. I had seen three not far from the road but quite the strangest sight was a large black swan waddling across the road like some fat dowager. The swan was not put off by the car horn and continued her sedate pace to the swampy patch on the other side of the bitumen.

I love the quivering and trembling of the hawks' wings in flight but in this early morning there seemed little movement over the great plains. Only a misty line shifting upwards as the frost rose. There was only the odd vehicle and we travelled the first two hundred kilometres so easily. I hate the distance that separates me from our sons and each time I leave Peter's property I feel a sense of loss. If it was only three or four hours' drive it wouldn't matter but it is too far for us to go just for a weekend now. If I was in my forties, or fifties even, it would be easier.

Back home there are nine messages on the answer phone and my world is as busy as ever. However, we both have a tan from the winter sunshine and feel refreshed. There is a call from my Hobart granddaughter to say that her semester report is on the way and that she is 'quite pleased' with it and hopes we will be too.

15

July

I am seventy-two today and I can't help reflecting on all that has happened in the past twelve months – a fiftieth wedding anniversary, one son's doctoral graduation, one grandson off to university, the other son's engagement, another grandson beginning life after IB with a move from Hobart to Melbourne, these and a host of other memories all crowd in.

Ian and I spent the day before at an art exhibition at the Mornington Art Gallery and then had a delicious lunch at the restaurant near the pier. Many years ago when Clarice Beckett paintings were being exhibited in large numbers for the first time, we had bought two. One was a small gem of a girl at the seaside (possibly Beaumaris), and the other was of a dreamy, misty landscape with an apricot-coloured background. They were not expensive at the time, although they now would do well at auction, but they have become part of our looking over many years, and always give us delight. We know the places that were familiar to Clarice Beckett and that adds to our pleasure whenever we drive around the bay. Perhaps I am becoming almost too knowledgeable about art. I know the paintings that are good and am able to see in one where the artist had painted with her lover, Percy Leason, because Ian and I have one of his paintings that I am sure was done at the same time. In both paintings you could actually trace the strong dark lines of his lampposts, although of course in the Clarice Beckett they were not so firm. But it was always good to see paintings and there were two other exhibitions, one with Hugh Ramsay, who had died all too young, and another by the not so well-known Jean Bellette.

The sun was turning the water silver, there was a group of retarded youngsters learning to sail just below us in the restaurant and our meal was served by a West Indian waitress for whom nothing was too much trouble. Quite close to the table a fat sparrow waited for crumbs, seemingly unafraid of restaurant patrons. I remember someone saying once that if you want colours for a room just look at a tree, a flower, a bird. The sparrow had sat there for some time and I had been able to observe the moleskin colour of his body, the deep brown of the head feathers, the dark black beak, the black and white speckled breast. It was all there, waiting for an interior decorator to use: a cream or moleskin carpet, deep brown curtains, black sofa and so on. It would be ideal for a study. The ideas from nature are endless.

After lunch we drove back with the sun streaming through the windscreen, tumbling white clouds in the sky, a blue, blue sea and yachts out on the water.

We had celebrated a day early because last year while we were out friends had come and left gifts on the doorstep and I felt that it was ungracious not to be at home. But to go out was better after all. I had spent a great deal of time on my birthday receiving telephone calls from people enquiring about my health. It was kind of them, but just for today I am trying to forget all that has happened during the previous twelve months and all the losses of the past years, my daughter, our three grandchildren I never see. I want to concentrate on the fact that I am here and alive and giving thanks for that. Ian and I have been offered a writing project. At our age that in itself is flattering, and I think that if we did it we could have a celebratory holiday afterwards.

We had dined on rainbow trout yesterday, but for tonight I have marinated in mint, garlic and olive oil some lamb chops from our son's property. They are delicious.

I have thought a great deal about families. How different they all are and how I as the eldest had always felt so protective of my younger brothers and how I was expected to care for them when they were young. Now they are able to do things for me. One of my brothers came down to fix the tap in the front garden this week. Ian's polio hand makes these tasks difficult, although he struggles on and never complains, but my mother had been good at repairing things around the house, she could draw, and had artistic genes. My middle brother takes after her and it is a wonderful tonic to have someone in the family to help with repairs. With the children interstate, it is sometimes possible for us to feel very alone when things need to be repaired. I know there are hundreds of people in the same situation and I don't want to complain, but my brother repaired the tap with such ease and insisted that we call upon him more often when things need to be fixed.

I have been reading again M. Scott Peck's *In Search of Stones*. His book *The Road Less Traveled* has been read by millions but this one is less well known. I am not sure what to think about our parenting. Our daughter no longer has any contact with us and so her three children are not part of our life either. My daughter's husband wants to possess her and has cut her off from family and friends and it is useless trying to explain this to friends who had known our children as young adults. They simply can't understand. I had written to my daughter while in hospital to alert her to the need for mammograms, but even then there had been no reply. Death is so much easier than prolonged and unresolved grief. Scott Peck has children in their thirties. Our eldest will be fifty next birthday and I know that generation so well. It hasn't been an easy road for the Pecks but I read with some agreement the following:

> Our new daughter had hooks in us well before her birth. Although difficult as a very young infant, attending to her every need was as natural for us as breathing. She had been born to be loved by us, and we had been born to care for her. And so it was with our other children. And so it continued as they grew and their needs changed from diaper changing, to story reading, to camping, to driver education and college selection.
>
> Only now they don't want our caring. That is to say, they do and they don't. They want our admiration and gifts and money, but

they don't want us. They don't want any of our wisdom. Certainly they don't want any of our advice. They also don't want to hear our stories. Partly that may be because they suspect some word of advice to be hidden in our stories even when it isn't. And partly it's because they're simply not interested. They have their own lives to live. They do want us to be interested in their lives, as long as there's no hint of desire to help, much less control. But at this point they really couldn't care less about our lives. In a sense they want us to like them but not to love them any more. And sometimes, even though they're our own children, it's not easy for us to like them when they're so different from us, when they no longer want our concern, and when their desire for our liking is so much of a one-way street.

Am I feeling sorry for myself? Yes and no.

No, because I realise that, in a way, they need me to stop loving them since I do not yet know how to love them without caring for them, without wanting the best for them so desperately that I slip now and then into advice offering. I have not learned to love neutrally. Maybe I'm starting to learn. I don't know. Maybe is the most optimistic I can be at this point.

But yes, I am feeling a bit sorry for myself – and for Lily – because it feels a bit unfair. I'm not saying that it is unfair. To the contrary, I think it is simply the necessary way of things. But that's my head speaking. On an emotional level it feels heart-rending. It feels unfair that God should have called me to passionately love my children for thirty years and now, rather suddenly, should be calling me to a rather neutered kind of love. It feels like I must almost *stop* loving them.

This is exactly how I feel about my daughter. After two sons I couldn't believe that I was given a daughter. And I still can't stop loving her. I don't think Scott Peck's words apply to my sons in quite the same way. But my daughter causes me greater anguish than I would ever have dreamt I would have to deal with.

16

I went to see my GP this morning. Arimidex may sometimes cause joint pains and my knees have been painful for some weeks and I thought that before I tried acupuncture it would be advisable to talk to my GP about it. He was encouraging. Said that I should 'give it a go', that joint pain came with the drug in some people and that if necessary to take Panadol in the first instance.

It is so frustrating when you aren't sure just what the tiny white Arimidex pill is doing to your system. Some days I feel as if I have a permanent hot flush with the cold weather having very little effect on me. I have tried taking the pill just after dinner at night but I frequently wake at two a.m., something I have never done before. But it is a powerful drug and I can only hope that it is keeping any cancerous cells at bay. I am sure that there are times when my husband isn't quite sure what to say or do when my emotions swing seemingly without any warning. For both of us the past year has been one of the most difficult in our life together. I try so hard to keep positive, to keep optimistic, to be grateful for the simple things of life. My mind tells me that all will be well but emotionally I know I am very vulnerable and still at times without warning tears well up in my eyes. It was reported in the news that the number of women presenting for mammograms had increased since the news of Kylie Minogue's cancer. Scarcely a week goes by without some news about breast cancer. A friend had telephoned that evening and in the course of our conversation told me that her sister-in-law had been given six months to live and was dying from cancer and they had found the primary cancer in her breast.

Last week as part of an ABC series on DNA the program reported on a new class of drug that promises to transform cancer treatment. Apparently fifty years ago the cause of cancer cell growth was not understood. A cancer researcher in America, Mary-Claire King, told how she was confident that if she could get enough samples she was certain that breast cancer was the result of damaged DNA. Other researchers' assistance fell through and it was only after Nancy Reagan's breast cancer was announced that Dr King received thousands of telephone calls from women anxious to help. They gave her information about their family trees, family histories, and she began tracing their genes with blood samples from living family members. In 1992 she had a breakthrough, finding the region that contains the gene. She had narrowed the gene to a small part of one chromosome and she discovered that breast cancer had stalked some families for generations. She tested the DNA of two sisters and discovered that the DNA of one put her at risk, but not her sister. For four years King and her team of researchers worked non-stop and in the end where to find the gene was discovered by an arch rival. But although the genetic test was a great breakthrough this alone won't help many people.

While all this was going on, a Norwegian by the name of Per Lonning had frozen a sample of every cancer he had treated over the previous ten years. He knew that one day this information would be invaluable to a researcher. Today it has helped scientists see the great diversity in cancers. By 1997 scientists had produced a drug that was able to target the faulty section of a cell and stop it dividing in a patient suffering from an advanced form of a particular type of leukaemia. So the future is bright, but not for those in the final stages of the disease.

17

August

Ian and I are both Leos. We both lead in different ways, but we are strong personalities in our own way. It took me some time before I really saw the differences in our style of leading. And now it is Ian's birthday and we are going to the Dutch Masters exhibition at the National Gallery. It is a Friday just before the lunch crowd and we are able to move freely.

I always enjoy watching the reaction of people to a painting. Often they want to see the paintings that have been used to advertise the exhibition, and that is fair enough, but today I enjoy the easy responses of a group of teenagers there with their art teacher. They are working on a questionnaire so they look very intently at all the paintings. It is helpful to have jugs, vases, cruets and a beautiful table rug to give an idea of the wealth of the middle classes during this time. The East India Company was trading all over the known world and much of the wealth came from their spice trade.

Many of the paintings depicted Dutch life of the period and there were numerous landscapes with northern skies but as always with blockbuster exhibitions you are drawn back to several works that have about them a compelling reality. Our son has always said that the entry fee is worth it if you find two or three stunning paintings that will remain with you. And this was certainly true. I especially liked the Pieter de Hooch interior with a mother delousing her child's hair – *A mother's duty 1658–60*. There were two windows in the scene, with the play of light coming in from both directions, and the open windows in the far room took your eye outside to a tree in the garden. The two Frans Hals portraits and the Rembrandt *An Oriental* had an immediacy about them that made you feel as though you knew these people.

Great art, it seems to me, draws you in in the same way that a poem, a piece of music, a piece of theatre does. It isn't easy to define what it is that separates 'great' from 'good' but it is the mark of genius. I don't think that this exhibition will draw the crowds that came for the French Impressionists but a great painting such as Vermeer's *Love Letter* glows from the wall and won't be easily forgotten.

I can still remember the Dutch paintings we saw in the Michaelis collection in Cape Town many years ago. Then it was the first time I had seen a collection of Dutch masters all in one place and I can still remember the impact they made on me.

We took Ian's birthday lunch in the gallery restaurant and the menu thankfully had gluten-free dishes so he was able to enjoy his meal. The winter sun came onto our table by the window and it gave us time and space to reflect on the paintings we had seen.

The evening was occupied with calls from our grandchildren and our sons and I long to have them all at the dinner table again. Perhaps one day soon.

Ian and I are still so much in love despite all the traumas of life. We are sent a poem by an Adelaide woman who had read Ian's journey of faith and knows something of our relationship. It is a poem taken from a collection of the poet Shelton Lea who died recently. Ian gives it to me to read.

> i dream of the soft slide of light
> i dream of the soft slide of light
> across the down of hair on your face,
> of the one note samba of your eyes;
> of the swelling gentleness of your lips,
> and of the you that you commonly call i.
>
> i dream of giant butterflies
> winging over sea
> and washed rocks gleaming in the sun.
> i dream of the dun skies, city spread
> and you lying naked on a bed
> dreaming.

oh God i dream of the seeming wonder of being
alive
despite the dreamings of death.
i dream of rose blooming,
of fate never moving from its prescribed path.
i dream of weeds flowering, breathless, in autumn.

18

Patricia, who had been at school with me and then my bridesmaid, telephoned today. She was ringing from Cairns, where she was attending a conference. Some years previously, her firm had wanted to sell pearls from their pearl farm and I had suggested they try Makers Mark in Melbourne. Makers Mark had bought a considerable quantity of pearls from the company and according to my friend I was due a spotter's fee. I had never heard of such a thing, and in any case I had been pleased to know that my recommendation had been successful.

Some time later, when Patricia and her husband, Michael, heard that we were going to Germany to research the Lutheran school history, she suggested that we spend time with them in Athens, and then travel with them at Easter to Kastellorizo, the tiny Greek island closest to the mainland of Turkey. Why not?

Ian and I left the cold European winter behind us and it was twenty degrees when we touched down in Athens. Our first meal was at a tiny restaurant in central Athens and as we walked back to Patricia and Michael's flat at near midnight the traffic was as chaotic as it had been when we arrived, with horns blaring, motorbikes flying past and the whole of the city area ablaze with light.

Patricia and Michael were wonderful hosts and wanted us to experience everything, so the next evening we all went to Sunion to see the sun setting. All the wildflowers were in bloom, brilliant red poppies, yellow daisies and white and lilac flowers (I don't know what they were) covering the hillsides. The beautiful pillars of the temple of Poseidon were set against what looked like floating islands as the sun set. Groups of laughing French schoolgirls were busy looking for Byron's signature carved into one of the pillars.

Dinner was at a restaurant by a tiny harbour and we ate the freshest of fish served with salads. The next evening it was in a courtyard restaurant where we dined on stuffed vine leaves, moussaka, tiny meat and tomato balls, and succulent roast pork with vegetables and salads.

Patricia and Michael had already booked a tour to Delphi and Meteora and the flight to Kastellorizo on Easter Friday. So many Greeks travel at Easter that they wanted to be sure of a flight reservation.

I had never experienced so many different restaurants in successive evenings. That night we had a meal at Piraeus with the Australian ambassador and his wife. She was a good friend of Patricia's and we ate by the side of the water with a forest of masts nearby. There were girls selling gardenias and bunches of red and pink roses. Calamari, prawns, sardines, the marvellous Greek dips and fresh bread provided an unforgettable meal.

The Greek museums place their artefacts so carefully, giving each statue, each piece of pottery, each icon its proper space. There was an exhibition from Russia at the art gallery entitled 'The Gates of Mystery'. It contained icons, embroidery and jewellery and it was like walking into a series of dark caves containing the glittering, magnificent treasures, with recorded Russian Orthodox singing in the background. Most of the pieces came from Novgorod. Many of the church artefacts were of silver set with precious stones and much of the embroidery of icons had been done with metallic threads and the sheer beauty of it all left Ian and me without words. It gave a greater understanding of the Orthodox tradition before we attended the Palm Sunday service at the cathedral in Athens. It was full of high drama with the archbishop and his priests garbed in brilliantly coloured robes, the archbishop himself wearing a jewel-studded crown. As the four of us entered we had been offered a sprig of bay leaves by a saintly-faced woman and we lit our candles. I prayed as I always do for those I love and for the unloved and needy of the world.

We returned home after a walk to the restored Athenian Library with its great statues, many from the fourth century BC and earlier. I thought that some of them rivalled the *Winged Victory* in the Louvre.

Never a dull moment. The next morning we were off to Delphi and as soon as the bus had left behind the suburbs we were in an area of fertile plains where we saw a woman guarding thirty or so sheep and a man leading a donkey. It all seemed so leisurely after the bustle of the streets of Athens. As we climbed to Arachova, the snow was still on the mountains and yet again the wildflowers were a riot of colour.

Tourism had multiplied since our family visit in 1977 and the gallery at Delphi was crowded with visitors. We were pleased to retreat to our hotel where from the balcony we could see as far as the Bay of Corinth, its water shining in the far distance. Later in the day when the tourist buses had returned to Athens and the area was quiet, we returned to see again the Temple of Diana and the Gymnasium. By then the only sound was of a cuckoo in a nearby tree. At a monastery not far from the hotel we heard how priests and resistance fighters had operated there during World War II.

Kalambaka was our next stopping place and during the drive there the mountain ranges seemed to go on forever. The bus driver told us that Greece is one of the five most mountainous countries: they are Norway, Switzerland, Albania, Greece and Austria, in that order.

From the hotel the grey peaks of Meteora were just visible. I noticed that among the postcards in the hotel lobby there were some with the peaks floodlit. Michael and I decided to go and see for ourselves as soon as it was dark. Sure enough we were able to see what looked like something from a child's book of fairytales. Michael called Ian and Patricia and the four of us took a taxi. The closer we got to them the more impressive they became, with one massive rock striated, another plain, another pitted like Swiss cheese. The town was packed with people out walking or dining or simply marvelling at the extraordinary sight.

The following morning on our way up to the monasteries the town had not yet woken up, or so it seemed. We passed avenues of plane trees and then the climb began. The monasteries are perched on the edge of the Uluru-like rocks and look down across the valley to the mountains. Today, supplies to the monasteries are hauled up by ropes or taken up on the backs of donkeys. Once out of the bus there was a climb to the monastery and I envied the monk being taken up in a crate! There are beautiful frescoes and murals in the now largely uninhabited monasteries and there is an ancient circular kitchen with a cone-like roof containing old cooking utensils.

Ian and I have been travelling for six weeks and when we get back to the flat in Athens we have to pack for Kastellorizo. It is Easter Thursday and all over Athens the bells are ringing. We leave the flat on Good Friday morning at four-thirty for the airport. The weather is perfect for flying, first to Rhodes and then in a small Fokker to Kastellorizo. The runway is very small and from it you can see the coast of Turkey.

Patricia and Michael had bought a house on the island some years before. Michael's father had migrated to Australia from Kastellorizo, as had a number of Greeks. Most of them have a vitality and energy that makes them successful businessmen, but they are still attracted to the island home of their parents and grandparents. The house Patricia and Michael bought is three storeys high but quite narrow and it has been beautifully restored and from the upstairs room there is a clear view of the deep-water harbour where in the island's heyday seaplanes brought visitors. The four of us quickly showered and changed ready for the Good Friday services. The bells were already ringing out. That afternoon we had gone to the church and watched while mothers with their children decorated the *epitaphion* (the representation of the tomb), with freshly cut roses, geraniums, irises and carnations, some of which had come on the plane with us from Athens.

The bell tower was floodlit as we climbed the marble-dotted hill up softly lit pathways to the church. Inside the church it was hot with the innumerable candles. The chandeliers were giving off their light and two sailors and two soldiers stood either side of the *epitaphion*. The choir seemed to drone on for hours as babies fell asleep, occasionally were taken home. More candles were lit, the priest sprayed holy water, the air was filled with incense and men and women kissed the cloth representing the shroud: it was strewn with rose petals. A serviceman almost fainted.

I long for a gulp of fresh air. At last the priest in his mauve and gold vestments leaves his seat and there is action. A young lad has been standing in front of the epitaphion holding a cross on which there are three wreaths, the central one made of rosemary and orange blossoms. The army and navy men raise the *epitaphion* and the four young boys who have held the candles lead the procession and everyone follows them out into the windy night. I feel that I understand Zorba so much better. These people are all Dionysian. They mortify the flesh, clothing and jewellery are so important to them, feast days are central, but the meaning of much of the ritual doesn't concern them. They are happy just to be participants in the drama. I suppose that everyone is part of their particular culture, but the contrast between the two Easters Ian and I had been part of – Lutheran and Greek Orthodox – could not have been greater. I thought I understood the Lutheran tradition where body, mind and spirit all seemed to be engaged in worship. At church this morning the children all kneel before a cutout of the risen Christ, then as a sign of his resurrection appearance the whole church stamps their feet as if the stone is being rolled away (or at least that was how I understood it).

We took lunch in a vine-covered restaurant near the water's edge with the priest still in his church regalia and the island people mingling with some people from yachts moored in the harbour. Greek music almost drowned out conversation so after calamari, salads and freshly baked bread everyone got to their feet, the tables were cleared and moved and the dancing began.

It went on until late in the afternoon, when Michael decided to show us the ancient Greek writing from the time when the place was the site of a temple to Apollo. The red castle, Kastellorizo, was built by the knights going to the Crusades.

While we were walking back to the house, an enormous ferry arrived bringing Easter guests. It almost filled the harbour as the sound of church bells came down the hill. Everyone dressed in their best for the church service. The children arrived carrying ribboned candles. The packed church waited until the door of the iconostasis was flung open and the priest walked through it carrying the Easter candle and shouting '*Christos Anesti*', 'Christ is risen'. As the gathering walked out into the courtyard, the bells rang with such ferocity that I felt they would split the tower. At the same time, everyone was lighting their candles and fire crackers, and, to my horror, dynamite exploded with a thunderous sound. There is a tradition that if you arrive home with your candle still burning and make the sign of the cross with its smoke above your doorway, you will be blessed for the following year.

The evening meal is the traditional avgolemono soup (egg, rice and lemon in a chicken broth) and it was followed by cheese, olives and bread and the traditional red eggs were cracked. The last person to keep their egg whole has good luck. Patricia, Michael, Ian and I went to bed at two-forty-five, exhausted.

The next morning as the four of us walked around the village women were making or had finished making fresh-flowered wreaths for their doors. It was all very festive. A friend of Patricia's had invited us all to a spit roast of goat for lunch. We sat at a table by the water and were enjoying the sunshine when our party suddenly realised that the church service was at five-thirty. Another mad scramble to change. The resurrection readings from the gospels were given in French, English, Latin and Greek. The person who had read in Greek held the icon of the resurrection as people filed past. Later, in the courtyard, the women danced the traditional resurrection dance and a cup containing a sweet almond-flavoured liqueur was passed around. Home and our best clothes for the island's Easter feast in the hall. Michael in his usual generous way had flown in the prawns and crayfish from Perth in enormous bags for his island friends to enjoy and the tables groaned with food.

I had hoped desperately for a rest day but the following morning and afternoon visitors arrived and before the sun set Michael wanted to show Ian and me the island in a rubber dinghy. The wind had abated and the sea changed in places from aquamarine to violet; we could see the coast of Turkey and the distant mountains across the water, coves, caves, tiny uninhabited islets, men putting out their nets, and occasionally a visiting yacht.

At last an early night so that we could leave early for Kas on the Turkish coast. The sea was calm and as soon as we got there Michael hired a taxi to take us to Myra. It is thought that St Paul was there in 60 AD and the tomb of St Nicholas is there. We saw ancient murals and a superb amphitheatre with pieces of broken pillars lying in the long grass. There were marble heads in different stages of decay: I would love to have taken one home.

The seats at the table where we stopped for lunch were covered with colourful Turkish rugs and the waiter was happy to see us. There were shops in Kas glowing with a great variety of spices and in a rug shop Patricia bought a delicate silk rug for their home in Perth. The wind had sprung up and we travelled back across the water with the salt spray in our faces. It was exhilarating.

The plane for Rhodes left at three the next day and it was a perfect flying day. On arrival in Rhodes we checked in at our hotel and then went for a walk along the tree-lined streets with people selling lace, leather and woollen goods. As the day faded the lights in the cobbled street of the Crusader knights came on and the battlements were floodlit. I love the warm cream of the stone buildings in Rhodes, so very different from Kastellorizo.

Patricia wanted us to see Lindos, once the capital of the island, so the next day we were carried up to the castle on the backs of donkeys. I felt sorry for the patient animals but was glad I wasn't walking. The sea on one side as we climbed was postcard-perfect with again the spring wildflowers in bloom on the slopes. There is a great sense of history in these islands and we were delighted to stop on our return to Rhodes at a place where women were painting ancient designs on plates.

We spent another two days in Athens before returning to Australia.

Both Ian and I wanted time to digest all that we had seen. It had been such an insight into the Greek psyche.

As I reflect on all this, it seems as if it was only yesterday. It is strange in the first year after cancer surgery the way your mind works. Everything is more vivid and the past seems to contract into a small time frame.

19

It is my book club night and the group will be discussing their response to Michael Dutney's book *Playing God – Ethics and Faith*.

In his introduction he says this:

> Regardless of creed, advances in science and technology at the end of the modern era have made bodily life a constant test and stimulus to faith. Raising questions such as: What do I believe? What are my values? To whom am I responsible? Ultimately in whom and what do I trust? What should I do?

I hope the discussion will move from theory into practice, for most of the group have experienced the death of someone they loved deeply. How did they deal with it? In one chapter of the book the author writes that taking risks is part of life and that as human beings we take risks when we make choices. If our choices aren't the right ones we are nevertheless responsible for the consequences. Whenever we make a choice, there is the possibility that we will be wrong.

I had taken a risk with hormone replacement therapy, but at the time it seemed the right thing to do and my surgeon had recommended it after my hysterectomy. I think that these days both of us would have made different choices.

Will it never end? Scarcely a day goes by without some news about cancer. There is a whole new class of drugs now that are able either to stop or slow down the growth of tumours by restricting the blood supply that nourishes the tumours, but most are exceedingly expensive. Surely a mother with young children is more deserving of such a new treatment than someone of my age who has had a good life? I wouldn't want to be the oncologist having to make the decision about who would receive a life-saving or life-extending drug. All these are ethical decisions.

There are days when I feel totally confused about all the new therapies. Only this morning I read of the death of an Oxford don, Michael Gearin-Tosh, who in his book *Living Proof: a medical mutiny* published in 2002 told of his diagnosis with melanoma. He had been given six months to live in 1994. Gearin-Tosh was an expert on the Elizabethan poet, Andrew Marvell, and had been tutoring at St Catherine's College, Oxford, for about thirty-five years. He was not impressed with the survival statistics for those undergoing chemotherapy and had decided on alternative treatments. With his regime of vegetable juices, injections, high-dose vitamins, coffee enemas and Chinese breathing exercises as well as using visualisation of his immune cells attacking the tumour, he had lived for another eleven years and did not die of the disease but of a blood infection.

I found it all very unsettling. Did I want to spend the rest of my life focusing on my health as he had done? I certainly watch what Ian and I eat and believe it to be a healthy diet, but is it enough?

When Michael and Patricia were visiting Melbourne after our trip to Greece, they said that they would like Ian and me to write Michael's biography. I said that we knew about biographies and it might be the end of our friendship, as it was a fairly difficult task to portray the life of someone close to you. Just as sitters are frequently unhappy when their portraits are painted, so it is with commissioned biographies. Ian and I finally agreed, because it seemed to us that Michael was typical of all those West Australians who had been at the forefront of the state's extraordinary development in the seventies and eighties and not a great many of their stories had been documented.

Michael had never kept diaries, there were no proper archives and the business was still expanding. We thought it would be a challenge. Patricia and Michael invited us to stay with them while we were working and we made their home our base while we travelled to see different aspects of the company. Our first visit was to Dongara at the end of the crayfish season. Michael had started there in a tiny factory and Patricia had practised as a GP for the district. The business had expanded to Exmouth Gulf and a prawn fishing enterprise that now sends prawns all over the world. Patricia had lived with their small children and Michael at Learmonth until the business was well established.

Ian and I watched with fascination while the girls in the factory removed the feelers from the tiger prawns before they were exported to Japan. Michael was always dreaming of new projects and his shipbuilding enterprise resulted from the necessity for more and more prawn boats. Michael was also fishing in the Gulf of Carpentaria. He had spent his early years in Darwin before they were evacuated during the Second World War and the north had great appeal for him. It wasn't long before he was starting up a pearl farm in the Buccaneer Archipelago.

It was necessary to visit the different arms of the company, but also necessary to get a feel for the distances between towns up the long Western Australian coastline. With modern technology as it is today, it is hard for the young to conceive of the 'tyranny of distance'. It was fortunate for the family and for their workers that Patricia was a doctor, but driving to Dongara and to Learmonth with a young family could not have been easy. Fortunately the family had all moved to Perth before the pearling began and light planes were flying all over the country.

Ian and I spent time at Cable Beach before taking a six-seater Cessna to the company's pearl-cleaning boat. That in itself had been an adventure. The spare part for the seaplane that was to have taken us from Broome to the farm didn't come up in time so the Cessna landed at Cockatoo Island. From there we were taken to the water's edge in a Land Rover, rolled up our jeans and waded out to a dinghy that bumped us out to the pearl-cleaning mother ship. The giant *pinctada maxima* shells that produce the lustrous pearls need to be cleaned continually and the boat sits in marvellous clear water renewed by king tides. It is a pristine world of red oxide cliffs and blue water with terns and dolphins coming close to the boat.

On a later trip, accompanied by Patricia and Michael and some Perth friends, we went by dinghy to isolated beaches with the purest sand and warm rock pools, and had meals on a beach that felt as if it was somewhere yet to be discovered. I felt I was too old for a jet ski but had to admit that racing through the water back to the mother ship afterwards was exhilarating.

The first time we went to Broome we were there for the pearl harvest and so were able to see the sorting room. The pearls gleamed yellow, gold, silver and apricot in a room flooded with light to help the girls grading the pearls on long trays. Occasionally an especially beautiful pearl would come up and there would be gasps of delight as it was passed around for everyone to see. The young women come up from Perth for the harvest each year and obviously enjoy the experience. The pearls are sized, sorted and polished with corn chips that give off a wax. These beautiful pearls have a ready market overseas and once this project was well established Michael was off on his next adventure. This time it was tuna farming in Port Lincoln.

At Port Lincoln Michael had supplied feed to the tuna fishermen. There had been tuna fishing in Port Lincoln since 1939 and still in the 1980s much of the tuna went to the canning industry. But all this was to change when it was found that tuna for sashimi could fetch $13.50 per kilo whereas canning brought them only $1.20 per kilo. It is possible to tow the fish very slowly from the Great Australian Bight to Port Lincoln, where they are placed in giant pens in the bay. There they are fed daily and rapidly gain weight.

Ian and I got up early to watch the fish being harvested. The boat was small and there was little protection from the bitterly cold wind once we had left the shelter of the harbour. We watched as the tuna were landed thumping and tossing on a rubber mat where they were killed quickly, gilled, gutted and placed into a slurry of ice. At every stage the fish were treated carefully and gently. We had left the wharf as the sun rose and it was early afternoon when we returned. The fish were unloaded from the boat into waiting trucks and taken to the factory.

Here we watched them being cleaned, blow dried and placed into long cardboard cartons for the journey to the markets of Osaka and Tokyo.

Patricia and Michael were great benefactors to Western Australia and while Ian and I were writing Michael's biography, *The Captain's Grandson*, Michael was much involved with the building of a replica of *Duyfken*, and it became a large part of his life. Indonesia, the Netherlands and Australia were all involved in the project. The hangar for the vessel was by the water not far from the company's office in Fremantle.

In 1605, the year de Quiros thought that he had discovered the great south land, part of the United East India Company's Feet was a *jacht* or lightly armed ship called *Duyfken*, or *Little Dove*. Because she was a smart, fast little vessel, she was chosen for a voyage of discovery the following year. Under the command of Willem Janszoon and with a crew of just twenty, they had nosed into the sand of Australia's Cape York Peninsula believing it to be the coast of New Guinea. Janszoon had found what was later to be named the Pennefather River.

Michael found all this exciting, watching the *Duyfken* take shape in the huge hangar at Fremantle, seeing the eager schoolchildren on the platform observing the workmen using traditional tools and methods to build the ship, and on the day of the launch no one was more proud as the little boat was lowered into the water on a perfect summer morning.

Michael died just before the book was launched at the University of Western Australia. Ian and I were pleased that he had seen a copy of the book before he was taken into intensive care. He had lived the same number of years as his grandfather, who had been such a role model for him.

Writing the biography had not only offered us beautiful landscapes but we had met a host of fascinating people; cray, tuna and prawn fishermen, boatbuilders, office managers, factory workers, pearling operators, and shop assistants.

21

Today as I write the sun is streaming in through the windows and I love every minute of living. Only this morning I noticed the new growth on the pruned roses, the masses of camellias flowering in the garden and there are two tiny finches on the bare branches of the blossom tree. I don't want to take anything for granted. Perhaps that is the gift that cancer gives. You take nothing for granted any more. But there are days when I feel totally confused about all the new therapies.

It is Daffodil Day for breast cancer today and the greengrocers had large buckets of them with some of the sale money going for research. I just couldn't buy any. I wanted to, but I knew that even as I arranged them I would be reminded yet again of all the women caught up in the nightmare of waiting for pathology results or buying a scarf to hide their bare scalps.

Ian and I had wanted to see the film *Look Both Ways*. Not just because we admire William McInnes's acting but also because his wife, Sarah Watt, had both written the script and directed it and it seemed an interesting theme for a husband and wife to explore together on film. The film deals with life, birth and death, and forces film-goers to assess their own responses to those times in life when the normal flow of living is suddenly disrupted. It could have been a 'heavy' film but because of the skilful script writing there are moments that lighten everything up and you find yourself laughing. One such moment was when a single dad is walking through the South Australian Art Gallery with his two children and the little boy mimics a crucifixion; flinging himself down to the floor, he lies there with his arms outstretched.

The characters are so believable and when Nick (William McInnes) is diagnosed with cancer and tells his journalist colleague, Andy's immediate response is 'You mean cancer cancer?' as though it could not be possible that Nick is ill with cancer. And of course friends don't know how to respond. The diagnosis does, however, give them all a reality check on their own lives. It all depends on 'where you are coming from', as people will say.

I cling to the rapid images at the end of the film that depict a bright outcome for the characters. One film critic has described the film as 'subtle, touching and thoughtful' and admired the way 'Watt has the capacity to show the way people think'. It must be one of the best of the current crop of films that seem to be heralding a renaissance in the Australian film industry, films like *Oyster Farmer* and *Three Dollars*.

More reports on cancer research and an article that advises people with cancer to search for available treatments on a website that lists more than sixty clinical trials for cancer. Another report published online by the British Medical Council found that high stress levels in women were found to decrease the risk of breast cancer. A Danish research group had asked nearly seven thousand women to rate their personal level of everyday stress and then followed up some eighteen years later. They found that those with high stress levels were sixty per cent less likely to develop breast cancer than those with low stress levels. All of this goes quite contrary to the current idea that stress increases the risk of cancer.

You find information in the strangest places. I was interested to read in of all things an article on elephantiasis a clear description of the lymphatic system. Because the lymph nodes are involved and one of mine was cancerous and the surgeon had removed all thirteen of them in the cluster, it was inevitable that my whole body would be affected. The lymphatic system maintains the balance of fluids in the system.

> It comprises a network of tiny tubes that reach into every part of the body, carrying white blood cells or lymphocytes in a clear watery fluid known as lymph. There are 600 lymph nodes in the body, small organs that cluster under the arms, in the groin, neck, chest and abdomen.

In some small way I feel more in control of my body's health the more information I have. This may not be for everyone, but it is for me.

22

Much has been written about what goes on in our minds as we sleep, and the pattern of our dreaming sleep has been divided into REM (rapid eye movement) sleep and NREM or orthodox sleep. I was sometimes able to recall a dream the next day, but not all that often. I was, however, aware of the strange workings of my mind during sleep. There were mornings when I woke up feeling refreshed, as if I had spent the whole night with my mind in a pleasant place. But this was not always so and last night my dreams left me feeling tired when I woke up.

As I changed the bed sheets, I caught the valance with my foot and then couldn't lift the mattress and straighten it at the same time. I felt angry. Angry that I could no longer manage things on my own as I had in the past. I didn't want to bother Ian to come and help with such simple everyday things, even though he was only too happy to help. I was the problem. It was my wretched independence.

Ian and I had decided to get another power point put in the study. There seemed to be extension cords everywhere and I was afraid we would fall over them. The young electrician who came is part of a great team of electricians we have had over the years. The house is on a slope so it wasn't difficult for Roger to get under the house. When the work was finished, we offered him a cup of coffee and as we sat drinking he commented on a picture of the campo in Siena hanging on the kitchen wall. I asked him where he had travelled and before long it all came tumbling out. He had grown up in Whyalla in South Australia and attended a school run by the Christian Brothers. The Brothers had an exchange program with a school in Calcutta and were always telling the students that they needed to make a difference, to leave something behind in life. After he had completed his studies and was a qualified electrician, Roger offered his services to an aid agency. He went with the agency to Romania, Albania and Calcutta, seeing things that changed him forever. Embalming small children, seeing handicapped children in institutions where they had been cramped for years and coming to a realisation that when human beings are deprived of life's necessities they will do almost anything to survive. The experiences had left a mark on him, changed him for ever. He told Ian and me that people were always telling him to write about his experiences but life was too busy. He is to be married in five weeks. Perhaps his wife will encourage him to write.

It was a good visit and came at just the right moment. It took away any self-pity I was feeling and put my own situation into perspective. The day was not the same after his visit. Something similar happened a few days later when our ancient washing machine decided to stop in the middle of a load of towels. Our electrical store arranged for their mechanic to take a look at it. He was an elderly Italian who had worked with washing machines for many years. He said that he was 99.9% sure that it was the motor. Did we want to replace the motor or get a new machine? We had recently bought a new refrigerator to replace the very elderly model we had. I was worried that in the middle of a heatwave it would suddenly die. The new model has some fine features to it, but was nothing like the quality of our ancient model. If a new motor would fix the washing machine I would prefer it. The old man was warm, courteous and totally charming. He would be back in two days with the new motor. Bruno was another human being who had not been caught up in the epidemic of 'affluenza' and just enjoyed his work.

My knees have been so painful of late that my GP thought there would be no harm in finally trying some acupuncture. Thirteen per cent of women on Arimidex develop painful joints and no doubt there was some arthritis there to begin with. I had never been involved with alternative therapies before but my knees are making me feel like an old woman so I took up my GP's recommendation and went off for a consultation. I knew that over the years I had not taken much care of my physical frame. I ate and slept well, but I am a physically shy person, really, and the thought of acupuncture didn't have great appeal.

I was ushered into a modern, architecturally splendid room and my massage began. I had not experienced this, and in any case I had always thought of massage as a pleasurable experience. On television patients were always being observed relaxed and in a dream-like state after a massage. With my lymph nodes removed from under my arm the masseur told me I was retaining too much fluid in my legs and he would work on them. I later learn from my GP that this was a most unlikely cause. I didn't think I was a wimp where pain was concerned. I don't mind the dentist but I found the pain of the massage almost unbearable and it went on for over an hour. After that, the acupuncture needles were applied. They were not a problem at all but I didn't feel like dropping off to sleep.

I was told to go to the local pool twice a week and to undergo a detox diet for seven days. I hadn't been to the local pool since my grandchildren were small and didn't want to spend two half days a week walking up and down in the water. Time was too precious. Did I really have a choice if I wanted to improve my health?

The diet was to remove the toxins in my system and as I looked at the list of forbidden foods there seemed very little that I could eat. I was already watching everything on Ian's coeliac diet and didn't want yet another problem with food. I knew that mine was an acidic system and that my preference had always been for tomatoes, lemons, spices and in fact just about everything that I had to avoid for a week. There would be a fifty per cent improvement according to the acupuncturist, but that would be after four more expensive treatments and the diet regime. I had invited friends for lunch on two days of the following week and Ian and I had been invited out for lunch in two days' time. Would it really make a difference? Perhaps I would just take Panadol as the GP had suggested. Ian and I went off to the supermarket together looking out for foods without wheat, rye, oats or barley for Ian and the few items I could eat if I went on the diet. No one had thought to mention to me at the time that the body's fluid balance would be affected after my surgery. I might have expected it if I had thought about it, but there were too many other things to be concerned about at the time.

Ian does his exercises for his polio leg in the morning and at night and I would have been happy to do any number of exercises, but to give up two half days for what would not be a cure seemed a waste of time. For the first time since my surgery I was angry. Angry with my body and angry with myself that while I managed Ian's fairly recent diagnosis of coeliac disease the thought of any diet for me that isn't absolutely necessary fills me with despair. I want to keep physically healthy and have my mind full of positive thoughts but I can only be as I am. I know that other people might see things differently. Cancer can't change who you are. To withdraw into a world dominated by concern continually for my physical well-being was asking too much of me at this stage. I thought I would ask my oncologist about it in a fortnight and take it from there. Was I being difficult? I hope not.

23

A telephone call from my university grandson who is studying ecotourism to say that one of his lecturers is going to put up one of his essays on the website. He is delighted. When he was in Year 12 he had revised his environmental science with me and our relationship has always been a good one.

The following morning there was a call from Paris. Our second son had just returned from Copenhagen and was eager to tell me all about his experiences with the charming Danes. Of course mentioning to people that he was a Tasmanian in the land of Princess Mary was a help. He and his partner were struck by the serious, stylish, hospitable and fun-loving people. I had suggested to him that they might visit some of the places we had so enjoyed all those years ago, but of course things change and the marvellous fish market with the fishwives in their splendid hats had moved and all that remained was a piece of sculpture depicting one.

It was a good start to the day. His son, our eldest grandchild, is still uncertain about his future. He is now in his third job since arriving in Melbourne. This time he is working as a waiter in a pleasant restaurant but some mornings his shift begins at six-thirty and although he hasn't been late yet, I know how much he hates the early mornings. He can't decide just where his future lies and as with all very bright students he could probably cope with most courses of study if he felt passionately about any of them. As with so many things as a grandparent it is a matter of exercising patience and standing aside rather than interfering – a sore temptation for most grandparents.

They came out for dinner tonight and both he and his partner are managing the transition from Hobart to Melbourne so well and he was looking fitter than he had for many years. Waiting in a restaurant is physically demanding but that is good for him and at the same time he has brain space to contemplate his future. 'They don't prepare you for life after Year 12 when you're at school, Grandma.' So he is learning what it means to budget. It is a temptation for all grandparents. They want to make life easier for their grandchildren, but I know that this unfortunately doesn't build character. Ian and I will help them with essentials if they can't manage, but I can see that our grandson has a real sense of self-worth, bringing in money for rent, tram fares and so on. Of course there is no such luxury as a car or even a bicycle at this stage. But it is still early days.

Our eldest and his fiancée have set their wedding date for November and Ian and I are delighted. Peter is so much in love and there is so much joy in his voice when he rings us. Like his father, he is a total romantic and wants a copy of the poem his father had published many years ago. He has remembered some of the lines in it and wants to send it to his love.

You smile.

And birds in my heart swoop singing
sanctus sanctus, sanctus

they swing and jest
over these leaping hills
Christus natus est
and so is love

fear is dazzled out of sight
by flashing wings
the clean cry of white
and freedom's chains
and birds in my heart swoop singing
sanctus sanctus sanctus.

Ian and I were taken out for lunch today by a friend who has had rheumatoid arthritis since she was in her thirties. She is a marvellous example of someone who has never felt sorry for herself, who struggles even to get dressed each morning and who regularly gives dinner parties and birthday parties for her friends. After lunch we all went for a drive out to Warrandyte and the wattle was blooming along the river banks. The gardens in Melbourne are a riot of colour at the moment with rhododendrons, azaleas, magnolias, blossom trees of various kinds and my favourite, freesias. At the moment, the few that are growing in the garden I have picked and put in a vase with daffodils and lemon rhododendrons. I could leave them in the garden but they are filling the dining room with their scent and each time I pass them I have the perfume of spring. Someone suggested to me recently that we should have five seasons as the Aborigines have, in which case this time would not be spring, but rather a season like pre-spring… In my opinion four seasons are only right for the northern hemisphere.

24

This weekend there was yet another article on cancer in *The Australian*. It reported on a convention in Orlando, Florida, the world's biggest annual cancer conference with twenty-five thousand participants. During the conference one of the speakers, Ian Smith, was the leader of the British group of doctors and head of the famous Royal Marsden Hospital. There was talk again of Herceptin. Herceptin interferes with one of the ways in which cancer cells divide and grow. Professor Smith said that a natural body protein sometimes attaches itself to another protein on the surface of breast cancer cells and this is what makes them divide and grow. Herceptin 'blocks this process by attaching itself to the HER-2 protein so that the epidermal growth factor cannot reach the breast cells'. Another speaker told his audience that 'we're approaching a point in five or six years' time when cancer will become a chronic disease like diabetes or blood pressure', but not everyone agrees with him.

The British journalist, Kate Carr, who died of breast cancer last year, had written in her book *It's Not Like That, Actually*, published after her death, because so much 'absolute rubbish was talked about cancer' it had made her journey that much harder for her. Scientists hope to increase the survival rate of people with breast cancer from eighty-four to ninety-four per cent. According to the newspaper article, 'one in three people in the industrialised West will contract a form of cancer in their lifetime'. Small wonder that people don't want to know about friends with cancer. Since 1975 cases of breast cancer and lung cancer have doubled. One fact that interested Kate Carr was that there are a dozen or more different kinds of breast cancer.

At the Orlando conference, Professor Bruce Ponder, who heads the Cambridge Oncology Centre in England, described cancer cells as lying low in the body and mutating until at some point they seize their prey, healthy cells and organs. Because there is a time lag between the cell change that damages the DNA it isn't easy to identify earlier traumas in patients which may have set off the cell change, and in any case the past is the past and part of life surely is dealing with the whole of it, not just the good, joyful parts. The conference seemed to reinforce the idea of the use of Herceptin in HER-2 positive patients. These tumours are aggressive and affect twenty to twenty-five per cent of the thirteen thousand women diagnosed with breast cancer each year. Researchers seem to think it has positive outcomes and it has halved the incidence of tumours recurring.

But Herceptin can cost as much as $60,000 for treatment. I think that in these circumstances people would sell anything to enable them to pay for the drug. So many of these new drugs pose questions for our society. Who will be able to afford them? Already Herceptin has been rejected by the Pharmaceutical Benefits Advisory Committee as not cost-effective and I sympathise with those involved in making the tough decisions on funding. It seems to me that there shouldn't be any discrimination when women's lives are at stake.

25

Our son's wedding plans are moving forward and he and his fiancée think that because there is so much work to do on the property in early November that perhaps they should wait until the autumn to have a honeymoon. What did Ian and I think? I know that the sensible, practical thing is to wait but the love they have for each other is so rare and, as I see life at the present time, you shouldn't wait for these precious moments. Seize them with both hands. Peter's fiancée has known the grief of a husband's sudden death and he the pain of divorce, and they are both mature enough to know that none of us is perfect. They accept each other's limitations quite happily. Their love is infectious for everyone around them, even when they are doing something as mundane as shopping in the supermarket.

What did they think about having a week in the South Island of New Zealand? Neither of them had ever been there before. Three years ago Ian and I had taken the Hobart grandchildren to the South Island for a holiday. We had chosen the South Island because when we looked at the brochures there seemed to be more dramatic scenery, more opportunities for adventure, especially around Queenstown.

The four of us get on really well in that strange way that happens when the passing on of genes seems to skip a generation. Our granddaughter is like me, the grandson the exact copy of Ian. The holiday had been a great success. We had punted on the river in Christchurch, taken a surrey with a fringe on top around Hagley Park with all four of us pedalling furiously. That day there was a World Busking Festival being held and we were able to watch a German juggler and a German escapologist. The Antarctic Museum provided more excitement with the Hagglund ride and we all had great fun walking through a simulated Antarctic landscape with the sounds of the roaring blizzard and extracts from Scott's diaries read from a recreated hut. Then we put on gumboots and warm anoraks and went into the freezing Antarctic room where the temperature registered minus twelve on the gauge.

In Queenstown we had taken a sky gondola ride to the top of Bob's Peak and the two grandchildren took the luge ride down. Then they had a ride with Grandpa (Grandma remaining on terra firma – the chicken) and hurtled down the Shotover River in a jet boat at speeds of about seventy kilometres per hour, spinning around 360-degree turns. The weather was so perfect that the twenty passengers all had a longer ride than usual, passing by me with the water spraying in their faces. Another evening we had taken a cruise on SS *Earnshaw* on Lake Wakatipu – a bit tame after the Shotover Jet, but we enjoyed every experience.

Bus journeys throughout the South Island were easy travelling through the mountains where *Lord of the Rings* had been filmed, and going through the fascinating Homer tunnel, a 1.2-kilometre tunnel that had taken twenty years to break through the rockface. At Milford Sound the weather was bright, although not sunny. The cruise on the sound takes you to the Tasman Sea and the water in the sound is so deep that it is impossible for the *QE2* to drop anchor there. Seals were lying on the rocks and the Bridal Veil falls had all the photographers busy.

The Franz Josef glacier is a mecca for climbers and even to walk along the lower edge observing that extraordinary blue as you walk along the rocky bed was a thrill for the grandchildren who had never seen a glacier before. On another day we had taken a bus tour into the Southern Alps and Mount Cook. There it was white and gleaming with the beautiful glacial river and the wildflowers reminding me of northern Scotland and Fort William.

For both Ian and me it was a holiday full of double delights.

The children had added to our own pleasure and we had established bonds that have been maintained ever since. It was small wonder that we thought our son and daughter-in-law-to-be would also enjoy it. When I was growing up my father had run a shipping company that managed *Wanganella*, a small liner by today's standards, but beautifully furnished. My father had often spoken of the beauty of the New Zealand countryside and since his first and favourite grandchild might travel there on his honeymoon seemed just right to me.

I do so need positive moments in my life just now. Today is the first day of spring and the birthday of my youngest grandchild. It scarcely seems possible but Ian and I have only seen her once, when we travelled to Armidale in a second attempt to restore relations with our daughter and son-in-law. I know enough about families to realise that most of them have things to deal with that cause them sadness and even despair, but for me the unresolved grief of estrangement from my daughter is often too much to bear. My daughter's little family know nothing of their grandparents, uncles and cousins. Every overture has been rebuffed and, after silent telephone numbers, their place of residence not listed on the electoral roll and so many other doors closed as a result of privacy regulations, I know now that it is possible for people to cut themselves off from the rest of the world, move interstate and only be found with the greatest difficulty. I know that part of it is brain-washing of the worst kind and not a day goes by when I don't think of my beautiful, talented and vibrant daughter. Strong and stubborn, she will manage, but at what cost? To use a word thrown about so frequently these days, there has been no 'closure' and there are days when the sharpness of my grief is terrible.

But fortunately today I can't dwell on it. I have old friends coming for lunch tomorrow. One of my favourite films is *Babette's Feast*, and as I prepare as much as I can the day before I am quite content putting orange segments into a Grand Marnier syrup to accompany my orange/almond cake. I make the chicken stock and then the soup and buy the salmon, leeks and tomatoes for the main course. Although there are three courses I will only serve small helpings and there will be a large salad. My friends and I all enjoy our meals but know how important it is to watch our weight. I excuse the three courses by telling myself that we only meet every eight weeks or so and three of them live alone now and only cook different courses for their families when they come to stay.

As with my piano playing, so with meal preparation. It is effortless for me and I have been cooking for so many years that I can make most things fairly quickly. I still cut out recipes from newspapers and buy cooking magazines trying out new ideas from time to time, but I have to confess to never having boned a leg of lamb. This week my young friend from Canberra is in Melbourne. She is an expert on boning a chicken and so I asked her if she had ever boned a leg of lamb. 'Not a problem,' she said. I marinaded it overnight and then placed it boned and flat and spread with rosemary and olive oil into the oven. Covered with baking paper and olive oil it didn't take very long, even though it had been a large leg. I served it to my grandson and his girlfriend with baked vegetables, cauliflower cheese and green beans. It was so easy to carve and beautifully tender and flavoursome.

Our granddaughter has arrived from Hobart for a week of her school holidays. She arrived in Melbourne having tried out a new colour rinse and at first I didn't recognise her. She has grown in the last three months and is going to be tall and slim like her father. Ian had spent quite some time on the telephone trying to get tickets to *The Lion King* and finally was able to get two from the local newsagency.

As we were having our first evening meal together Lily said, 'My friends all said, "Are you going to Melbourne to see *The Lion King*?" and I told them I was going to see my brother and my grandparents.' Ian got up from the meal table, opened the study door and brought down the advertising brochure and the tickets. She squealed with delight.

She is the sort of teenager who enjoys everything in life – playing Scribbage, going to the movies, shopping whether for food or clothes or even just helping prepare the evening meal. She put on her best clothes for *The Lion King* and we are sure it was the highlight of her visit. Ian saw her looking at all the T-shirts and other merchandise and although he could never be considered a shopper he bought her a keyring and a T-shirt which she wore on the flight home. I had spent a morning at a clothing mecca – shop after shop of clothes for all ages, and we came home with a new pair of jeans, a new top, a jacket and a white handbag. It was such a pleasure following her around the shops, watching her carefully appraising each garment and then looking at the price tag. My knees are so painful that a morning's shopping was about all I could manage. I am quite sure that the medication is causing the severe pain and I can scarcely wait to ask the oncologist about it next week.

26

There is some good news in Friday's newspaper that a natural compound found in simple things like cereals, beans and nuts have within them 'a potent agent for fighting cancer'. It appears that the compound in them not only inhibits the growth of tumours but helps in the treatment of the disease, may be taken in large quantities and is non-toxic. The compound is called inositol pentakiphosphate and is rich in such things as cashew nuts, peanuts, kidney, pinto and navy beans. Navy beans apparently are the beans used in cans of baked beans. Cooking increases the effect of the compound. It is suggested that the dose be three cups of beans each week. There was also good news for pre-menopausal women in the fight against cancer. For women in this group it appears that new digital technology is more effective in diagnosing tumours in the under-fifty age group.

With more women being diagnosed with cancer each year, there are more articles coming to the notice of the general public every week. At the University Medical Centre in Utrecht, Holland, scientists had studied twelve thousand healthy middle-aged women born between 1932 and 1941 and who were part of a breast screening program. They discovered that 'left-handed women are more than twice as likely to develop pre-menopausal breast cancer as non-left-handed women'. While all the causes of breast cancer are not yet known, every large study adds to the sum of knowledge of the disease and its prevention.

Even with all this information becoming available, it seems as if many people are reluctant to check out breast abnormalities. Three thousand women had been surveyed and only half of them knew that the risk of breast cancer increased with age. Perhaps the very word 'cancer' is too frightening for some women to deal with.

Ian and I have been subscribers to the Australian Chamber Orchestra for some time and find these young musicians playing with such skill and such energy leave us at the end of the concert with renewed vigour. But not tonight. It wasn't the playing, it was the fact that a concertgoer we have got to know there was in her seat for the first time in several months. Her hair had returned, but she had lost a great deal of weight and although the actual word was not used it was obvious from our conversation that she was still having chemotherapy each week. That same week we had met another friend of similar age undergoing weekly treatment. It seems to me that it is like an epidemic, but a silent one. I had watched Sigrid Thornton in the television production *Little Oberon* and admired her for being prepared to play a forty-five-year-old grandmother dying of cancer and having her hair shaved for the part. Anything that encourages people to have regular mammograms has to be helpful.

27

Another visit to my oncologist and it is, as always, life-enhancing. He thinks that quality of life is more important than length of life and I agree. I will go off Arimidex for three weeks and then go back to Tamoxifen.

It is now six days since I stopped taking Arimidex and I wonder whether it is just imagination that my knees are less painful. I have been on my feet all morning, the humidity is high, and it is still early days. It obviously has and effect on your system when you stop taking it. If only I was a scientist.

When we were doing research in Perth and travelling to Fremantle most days we often saw the ferry leave Rottnest Island and we had promised ourselves that one day we would take a day off and travel the short distance to the island. But of course it had never happened. Rottnest is a great place for school leavers to let their hair down at the end of Year 12 exams. There is news from London that there is a rare coral found only in the sea around this island that is able to produce a chemical a hundred times more potent than the anti-cancer drug it mimics. As yet no one knows why it is that this particular coral produces eleutherobin but it is part of the coral's defence system. It will greatly assist people who currently use Taxol to treat their breast, ovary or lung cancers. The article states that 'eleutherobin works by interfering with mitosis, the process by which cells split apart and divide. It has been found to be effective against 20 to 30 different cancer cell lines and scientists hope that an artificial form could be even more powerful.'

My natural curiosity prevents me from ignoring articles on cancer research, and sometimes, as in a newspaper today, there are helpful suggestions for ways to alter the risk of cancer. A cancer epidemiologist has discovered that if women have two copies of the alanine gene they are generally four times more likely to have breast cancer than those with a 'valine variant'. I don't know about these variables but if pre-menopausal women eat lots of fruit and vegetables the risk goes down substantially. Of course diet alone can't fight cancer but food rich in anti-oxidants is obviously a help. The health of cells, however, is obviously dependent upon a whole range of things.

For my granddaughters there is the hope that with technology racing ahead it will be easier to detect the first sign of a cancer developing. It is forecast that in the next ten to fifteen years a woman, wherever she is, on a cattle station in the arid interior or in an inner-city apartment, will be able to check on the behaviour of a cancer-causing gene. All she will have to do is provide a blood sample for a nanoparticle-based DNA profiling test. That is, she deposits a drop of her blood on a plastic chip, seals it and inserts it into a reader attached to her desktop computer. The data the chip reveals is uploaded to a hospital and in seconds an analysis is forwarded to an oncological specialist. Later by video link, the specialist will discuss the results with the woman. Some brave new world, that. I admire the hours and hours of painstaking research going on all around the world in search of a cure, but there are certainly promising signs in many areas.

This morning there is a short piece in the paper saying that a British 'electronic music whiz' is hoping to become the first musician ever to use the sound of cancer in a dance track. It seems that the expertise will come from NASA via a scientist who specialises in recording cellular activity. Is there no end to it?

The chief executive officer of Breast Cancer Network Australia has just returned from the US and in Nicosia she led an event that brought together breast cancer survivors from Cyprus's Greek south and the Turkish north. It seems that women throughout the world are uniting to alert more and more scientists to the need for more and more research into this disease.

As I write things down in my notebook I think that I am really writing a life in twelve months. Every day is to be treasured irrespective of what the years ahead will be.

28

September

My brother has designed the poster for the Embroiderers' Guild spring exhibition and asks me if I would like to see the exhibition. As we walk around it, I know that I will never be able to produce the delicate work of some of the pieces, but they are so beautiful to look at and the embroiderers are leaving something behind in their imaginative work, whether it is a baby's shawl, a quilt, an embroidered garden or a beautiful flower. Some of the framed work would look just right hanging on a wall.

The best news of the week is that there is a letter from our son in Paris to say that he has decided to settle with his partner in Melbourne when they return in late October. Perhaps it is an acknowledgement that Ian and I won't be around for ever and he wants to see more of us and his son now living in Melbourne. Ian and I haven't had a member of our own family living in Melbourne for nearly twenty years and I can scarcely believe that there will be someone to support Ian. He is gardening today and although I weeded for a time I know when to stop now but I hate leaving Ian to complete the job. The garden has never looked lovelier with so many plants in full bloom. This morning I picked two armfuls of flowers to take inside and you couldn't see where they had come from.

Plans are now well advanced for our son's country wedding. Ian and I could write a book about the weddings of our two sons and daughter. I think the necessary phrases are 'be flexible' and 'go with the flow'. It was certainly necessary for the three earlier weddings and I would never have predicted the variety in a million years. What my father had made of them all I can't imagine, but I know he would approve of this one, for Peter was his first and favourite grandchild.

The first wedding of our three children had been at Warrnambool by the Hopkins River, where we all gathered in spring sunshine. The bride and groom were extravagantly dressed, their friends more casually, and the reception was at the TAFE college nearby. Ian and I had travelled down from Melbourne with the wedding cake in the back of the car, the minister wore a bright open-neck red shirt, and it was different from any wedding we had attended, but there have been many less traditional weddings since then with our friends and our friends' children. We did our best to fit in with the bride and groom's plans.

The next wedding was a very formal affair with everything planned well in advance. It was top hat and tails and the bride and her three bridesmaids looked beautiful. The old Anglican church was full of gorgeous flowers and the reception was in a beautiful club house and no expense was spared.

When our daughter's husband-to-be refused to be married in a church, our sitting room seemed to be a reasonable compromise. The celebrant, a family friend, was also an ordained minister and she conducted the ceremony with great sensitivity. Afterwards the guests all walked up the hill to the reception rooms. It was a perfect December day and our friends all accepted it as just another type of wedding. I had found it all a little taxing with my two sons, their wives and three small children travelling some distance to attend, the home to be decorated with flowers, the tulle from my wedding gown draped with roses on the stairs, and sufficient seating for the older members of the family. I suppose that all mothers have an idea at the back of their minds about their daughters' wedding days, especially if their two sons are already married. I had kept my own wedding dress. It was made so expertly by my Scottish great-aunt. I had hoped that one day my daughter might wear it. Ironically my daughter was almost an identical weight and height as I was on my wedding day, but when Jane decided against being a bride, I put it back in the top of the wardrobe, saying nothing but hoping that perhaps one day a granddaughter might have it altered and wear it.

This time it will be a country wedding in the late afternoon early in November. We have yet to meet the bride's extended family and I want to look just right. People are reluctant to admit it, but first appearances do matter, and for our son's sake I want to look my best. I rejected a tailored plum frock with a fine embroidered jacket with cream roses; it was gorgeous, but I knew that I would never wear it again.

How we continue on in the pattern set for us in childhood. I remember shopping with my mother when she chose her outfits for two of my three brothers' weddings (my mother had died before the youngest brother married). I was the one urging my mother to buy the beautiful clothes and even as I looked in shops for something to wear I wasn't sure whether I was weeping or raging inside that there was no daughter beside me to give me an honest answer as to what I looked like. I know that my emotions are not as they once were. Tears come all too easily. I don't want Ian to see them and do all that I can to prevent it. His daughter's absence sears him, too.

It is seven-thirty in the morning and there is a loud knock at the front door. Ian jumps out of bed and I hear 'Clothes dryer for Hansen.' 'I think you have the wrong address.' 'Hansen, 33?' 'Yes, that's right.' 'Well, this is for you, mate.' When we were staying with Peter he said that he hadn't felt a need for a clothes dryer until this last winter when the drought broke. He thought perhaps he should get one to be there for his new bride. In his generous, extravagant way he had bought one for us, too. I telephoned but he was already out in the paddocks and it wasn't until he returned at lunch time that I was able to confirm that he had ordered it. 'I couldn't bear the thought of you and Dad rushing out to bring clothes in off the line. You're too old for that now.' I know that soon I will be wondering how I ever managed without one, but until now it was never high on our list of priorities.

We have arranged for our grandson to see a careers adviser. He needs someone outside the family to convince him of his ability. He related well to the interviewer, did the Myers–Briggs test and to our great delight he has now enrolled in a university course with only days to go before applications close. He has had two years away from study of any kind and is missing the mental stimulation he needs to feel fulfilled. At the moment he is working two jobs in an attempt to save after paying off a loan. I admire him for his capacity to work and change. He frequently begins at six-thirty and there was a time when he couldn't manage to be at school on time even though it was only ten minutes walk away from his home. I remember one report that listed him as late twenty-eight times in one term. Strange things, genes. The test he took showed that he works best alone, is not a team player, but such a warm, attractive young man who I am sure will ultimately reach his potential.

My friend in Suffolk turns eighty this month and I was in despair of ever finding anything suitable to send when I discovered that the Museum of Contemporary Art in New York has opened a gift shop in Melbourne and their brooches and necklaces make wonderful gifts. Jeanne had been a wonderful friend to the family since we first met when Ian was teaching at the same school as her husband in London and we arrived there with our two pre-school sons. Each time we went to London on leave or en route to somewhere else, Jeanne and her husband welcomed us warmly and we had spent a marvellous summer holiday with them in a little village just outside of Bath, stayed with them when they retired to a village near Wells and were delighted to welcome their son to Australia. He married an Australian girl several months ago.

I have just finished reading Sebastian Faulks's remarkable novel *Birdsong* and knew from the very beginning of it that it would be, as the reviewer of the *Sunday Times* said, 'deeply moving'. Reading it as I often do, late at night, it frequently delayed sleep. It was all so intense and so closely entwined with my own life in a strange way. Ian's father had enlisted with the Army Medical Corps in World War I but found that he was unable to just look on and transferred to the infantry. He was with the 7th Battalion already in France, where most of the novel is set. Like Stephen in the novel, Ian's father had never talked to us about his experiences, although there was an extraordinary photo on his study wall of the bleak, shelled landscape where fighting had taken place. In World War II he was Chaplain-General for the other protestant denominations and had a rare understanding to bring to the suffering of others. Not only had he the experiences of war, but his young wife had died during World War II when Ian was still recovering from polio. As I read *Birdsong* and of the experiences of men in the trenches I knew why it was that so few were able to speak of the horror of it all.

My mother's life had been changed by war, too. My mother never told me, but I heard from my great-aunt that her father was unable to care for her when he returned from World War I and she had been reared by her grandmother. The trenches, the death of his young wife before their daughter's first birthday, all these things were too much for the young man to deal with. When her grandmother left for Australia to be with her widowed daughter and two granddaughters, she had no choice but to accompany her. She was a teenager and probably thought that one day she would return to the land of her birth. But she never did. It must have been a terrible grief. Now, a decade older than my mother was when she died, I wish desperately that she had felt free to talk to me about these things, but silence was her way of dealing with it. She had put a shell around the tender, painful parting from aunts, an uncle that she adored, and her friends. It was the only way to get through it all.

I am reminded of all those lost young lives from that war to end all wars when my grandson comes for lunch. He is tall, slim, with waves in his sleek, dark hair and looks just like the photo of his great-grandfather in army uniform that sits on top of the piano. I am sure they would have understood each other very well.

Our book group tonight is discussing a book by Thomas Moore,

Care of the Soul. It is an interesting read and I am particularly taken with the sentences 'There is a Job-like mystery in human suffering and loss that can't be comprehended with reason. It can only be lived in faith.' That it comes from the most personal part of our being I have already discovered. Moore goes on to say, 'We have to arrive at that difficult point where we don't know what is going on or what we can do.' I feel like that. Especially with the continual questions of well-meaning friends. 'How are you going?' I don't really know, and even after the mammogram next week I probably still won't know just what is going on in my body. There is a quote from Keats's *Endymion* that resonates with me.

> But this human life: the war, the deeds
> The disappointment, the anxiety.
> Imaginations, struggles, far and nigh
> All human; bearing in themselves this good.
> That they are still the air, the subtle food
> To make us feel existence.

When asked by patients, 'Do you think I'm on the right track?' Moore replies, '…the only thing to do is to be where you are at this moment, sometimes looking about it in the full light of consciousness, other times standing comfortably in the deep shadows of mystery and the unknown.' I agree with him when he writes, 'I suppose one of the gifts of illness is that you have time for reflection, of non-doing.'

There is a delightful article in today's paper written by Richard Flanagan. He describes watching his mother knead the dough for bread in the Tasmanian home of his childhood. A simple act, but a gift she passed on to at least one of her six children. Even as I read the piece the world seemed to slow down, waiting for the yeast to rise in the dough. The process can't be hurried and it isn't like the new modern breadmakers loved by modern housewives. Like so many important things in life it needs to be given time.

I remember when Ian first fell in love with Persian rugs, and when we bought our first many years ago. The grandchildren were still very young and we made a game out of looking for mistakes in the intricate patterns and designs in the rug. Living with the rugs intimately over several decades now, giving time to reflect on the young weavers and the ancient craft has added great quality to our daily lives. At night when the lights are off and subtle, the rugs gleam like jewels on the floor.

In his book, Moore emphasises the simple nature of things like washing dishes, putting clothes out on the line, weaving, knitting. So many little epiphanies waiting to be experienced. The American poet and novelist John Updike observes the simple sight of washing on a clothesline in his poem *Wash*, and the last two stanzas read,

> From an upstairs window it seemed prehistorical
> Through the sheds and fences and vegetable gardens.
> Workshirts and nightgowns, long-soaked in the cellar,
>
> Underpants, striped towels, diapers, child's overalls,
> Bibs and black bras thronging the sunshine
> With hosannas of cotton and halleluiahs of wool.

In a delightful poem entitled *The Broad Bean Sermon*, Les Murray describes the infinite variety of beans growing in his garden and partway through the poem he reflects on the wonder of the ordinary.

> Going out to pick beans with the sun high as fence-tops, you find
> plenty, and fetch them. An hour or a cloud later
> you find shirtfulls more. At every hour of daylight
>
> appear more than you missed: ripe, knobbly ones, flesh-sided,
> thin-straight, thin-crescent, frown-shaped, bird-shouldered, boat-keeled ones,
> beans knuckled and single-bulged, minute green dolphins at suck.
>
> beans upright like lecturing, outstretched like blessing fingers
> in the incident light, and more still, oblique to your notice
> that the noon glare or cloud-light or afternoon slants will uncover
>
> till you ask yourself Could I have overlooked so many, or
> do they form in an hour?

Moore suggests that the arts practised at home nourish us because they foster contemplation when we are doing the household tasks of cooking, arranging flowers or doing repairs.

I have often wondered over the past months why I have set down my thoughts and feelings and think that Moore provides me with an answer when he writes, 'To the soul the past is alive and valuable and so is the future. As we perform the alchemy of sketching or writing upon our daily experience we are preserving our thoughts for those who follow us.' I know that I am trying to capture the eternal in the everyday.

Researcher-journalist Hugh McKay quotes from Muriel Dumont of Louvain University in Belgium. She is writing about the fear of terrorist attacks that is gripping the world and the way in which we respond to fear: 'the natural tendency when afraid is to do whatever is possible to regain some control and protect oneself as far as possible from terrorism's dangers.' Defiance and anger is one way of taking control and becoming more powerful and optimistic, because anger is easier to deal with than fear. Another way is to be nonchalant, 'to whistle in the dark'.

McKay writes about the way we respond in our lives to any serious threat. I think that I responded to my cancer at times with anger, defiance and nonchalance, all three, depending on the day. Now that Arimidex is out of my system and I am back on Tamoxifen I feel as if I can manage. For me, Arimidex and the attendant side effects I had was a fearsome prospect, but I know that for the women who can't tolerate Tamoxifen it is probably a good alternative drug.

Our son and daughter-in-law-to-be are in Melbourne to buy the wedding ring, his suit, a shirt for one of his sons and to finalise the honeymoon arrangements for the South Island of New Zealand. They come home for lunch with half of the list attended to and our grandson, who is always happy to have some time out of boarding school, arrives with them for lunch. They have bought the grandson a vivid pink shirt (his choice), and he insists that the colour is 'pearl,

Grandma'. He puts on the shirt and tie with his suit and we all agree that he looks very smart. Peter, who hates the city, looks as though he would much rather be mustering a paddock of sheep than attending to all the details of the wedding, although he keeps looking at his love with such tender eyes.

I do enjoy their company. It is so much easier to forget about aches and pains when there is the wider family around. After lunch our grandson changed into work clothes and moved a climbing rose. It was in a large pot and it wasn't the best time to move it but it was too heavy for Ian to lift and our grandson moved it with so little effort that I was amazed. I forget how strong he is now and how much he does on on the farm in the holidays.

The following day, our son cut down a bush with similar ease. There was a time when Ian and I were not prepared to sit back and let someone else do the heavy work, but we still manage the garden without help, and the grandsons love to be useful whenever they come to stay. A year ago Ian and I would have struggled to do everything ourselves.

Ian is off to see the doctor this morning. He has an asthma-like cough that has gone on for too long and prevents him having a good night's sleep. I know that he is worried about my visit to the surgeon this week. The only other time he had a similar attack was in the spring in Devon when news came that his father had died. He can't bear to talk about it, but the brain and the body are in strange harmony, or disharmony. His body is reacting to his inner turmoil.

Love is a wonderful thing, but the symbiosis when two people are deeply in love can be a cruel thing if one partner is ill. I have tried to be tough throughout these past eleven months, but I am consumed with thoughts about the mammogram and the visit to the surgeon. Whatever I do to keep busy makes little difference. I feel so much for Ian, too. He is hypersensitive, a gentle and loving husband, but the minus side is the nearness of our thoughts – our dreads, our fears. This morning I watched two large ravens pull a young baby from the nest of a wattle bird in the garden. One of them took it to the top of a casuarina tree and proceeded to pull it apart. I think that my anger at the scene was too great until I realised that I was feeling as helpless as the young bird being devoured by the raven. A stupid thought, but true.

The GP sent Ian to a respiratory specialist 'just to be on the safe side'. I wait at home wondering what the news will be but he returns in two hours with good news. His lungs are fine, but the polio is rearing its ugly head again. This time it is affecting his breathing rate. Expiration is fine but he is not inhaling well and the weakness of the vocal chord muscles is evident. With all his lecturing and public speaking over the years they have had a fair workout, but I am still sure that much of it has to do with the stress of waiting for the mammogram results.

29

November

Here it is. Almost twelve months to the day since my insect bite, the first suspicion that something was wrong, the mammogram, the needle biopsy, the core biopsy, followed so quickly by surgery. Now the wheel has come full circle and I am about to have my first mammogram since the surgery. My stomach heaves as I try to eat breakfast. I know that if I just have coffee and orange juice, Ian will notice. I come out of the bathroom and put on my pink blouse and top. Whenever I wear this combination, people comment on how well I look and I need to feel good about my exterior, whatever is going in inside of me.

The radiographer is an elderly white-haired woman with a lovely smile. She knew just how to put me at ease and told me after the mammogram was done that there would only be a ten-minute wait. 'They are the longest ten minutes of your life, dear. I know.' So I sat in the cubicle and glanced at a magazine, trying to feel calm. The door opened wide and the dear woman said, 'Beautiful. You can get dressed now.' Not the dreaded 'I think we will just do one more', or 'we need one from the other side'. I am not sure that I have that much confidence in mammograms now, but it is the best way, whatever I think. Now there is only the surgeon's examination of my remaining breast after looking at the X-rays. In forty minutes it is all over. Not all over, of course. Not all over ever again, but over enough for me to get on with life and return for another mammogram in four or five months.

I feel so much more optimistic having weathered almost twelve months and I can look forward to the wedding and the joy of it all with a light heart now. It would have been terrible had I been forced to greet people and smile if the results had not been good. I am so thankful. I deal with most things these days by anticipating the worst and then anything else is manageable. I have lost one breast, I know the procedure, so if the other breast has to be removed it will not be a journey into the unknown this time. But all is well thus far.

There are certainly more positive than negative articles on cancer in the newspapers but the Saturday following my mammogram there is a rather depressing article which included a statement from an American epidemiologist who, amongst other things, said, 'Tamoxifen doesn't really cure it [breast cancer] but keeps it in check.' The same article reported that between twenty and fifty per cent or more of cancer patients are thought to use complementary medicines. I believe that the medical profession as a whole needs to be more open-minded in their approach to cancer. There don't appear to have been any really significant breakthroughs in cancer research in the past decade or so when millions of dollars have been given to it. That is not to say that discoveries haven't been made that may ultimately provide a cure, but until such time arrives there seems to be little doubt that often a range of treatments rather than one single approach is the best way to help women remain cancer-free after surgery.

Support for women seems to come from many areas, but the coordination of treatments that make a woman feel supported and confident is still rather haphazard. I am fortunate because I have had a husband and friends to help me manage the disease, but what about single women, widows, young mothers with children? How do they manage? Many people are working hard to make better outcomes for everyone, but I feel that there is still much to be done.

30

I have just come home from my school reunion. I'm not much into reunions but offered to be on the committee that had arranged the last one. It was so different this time. Five years can make a great deal of difference at this stage of women's lives. People are prepared to say how it is for them. At my table for lunch were two girls who had travelled the same bus route to school with me for some years. They know of my mastectomy and told me that they had had both breasts removed several years apart. One had opted for a reconstruction, the other had not. They had both 'moved on' after their surgery; one was still practising as a GP and the other leading a full and active life. If the ratio at their age is one in every eleven women with breast cancer, I wonder how many others in the room were in the same position. You could scarcely ask them to raise their hands.

They all seemed to be happy despite the usual upheavals that happen to women who left school five or six years after World War II. Happiness has a great deal to do with our immune system and scientists have discovered that when happy people are given a flu vaccine, they develop more antibodies as as response to the vaccine, and a study of one thousand Israeli men stated that those who were loved by their wives had a fifty per cent reduction in their angina and cardiac disease.

I reflect on my generation of women, most of whom had taken up careers again when their children were all at school, and they had juggled work and home and now were watching their daughters trying to do everything. Our daughters are often fearful that if they don't keep up some part-time work even when their children are very small, they will miss out on promotions, or even lose a recognition of their skills in a time of rapid change. Our role as grandparents has been so very different from that of our mothers.

At the end of the afternoon everyone says that the reunion has made them all feel younger as they recalled teachers, excursions, all those vivid impressions we store away.

I have so much going on in my life at the moment. I've been sent a piece of the material of the frock my future daughter-in-law will wear at her wedding on Saturday. I have been asked to do the flowers in the church and an arrangement in the reception hall, and I want the church flowers to match the colours in the bride's dress. Today is hot and steamy in Melbourne and I wonder how the flowers will travel in the car all the way up to the Riverina. I don't care for artificial flowers but I know that they often provide good block colour when mixed with fresh ones. At the same time I check with the florist and they will supply delphiniums, iris, and whatever else the market has in pale mauve and apple green.

My younger son and his partner invited us for lunch today. His partner had gone to so much trouble to prepare a delicious gluten-free lunch and we sat down to a risotto, salad and scrumptious ginger pudding with cream. They are house-sitting a Victorian terrace cottage for two writers who have gone to France for a few months. The weather is still in the thirties, but there is a breeze from the front door right through the long passage to the picturesque back garden and the house is a treasure trove of books and artefacts. They have brought back French perfume for me and a CD of organ works by Helga Schauerte-Maubouet for Ian; our son had heard her playing in the Lutheran church in Paris. They are such buoyant pieces, employing just the right stops for the arrangements of Bach, Albinoni, Telemann, Torelli and others.

It is so good to have David only a short distance away. I feel the sense of support he brings to Ian. This last year has placed an enormous strain on him with no immediate family in Melbourne. There have been days when I'm sure I haven't been easy to live with. There were days when nothing in the daily routine seemed important, and yet the strange thing was that while I was busy doing these mundane tasks I found myself able to move on from the low moments and be optimistic about the future.

There are always strange discoveries being made in medicine. I am preparing a chicken curry for dinner tonight. I read recently that circumin, the spice that is the main ingredient in turmeric and the source of an Indian curry's yellow colour can stop breast cancer spreading to the lungs. At the same time it increases the effectiveness of Taxol, 'the frontline drug against breast cancer'. Trials of circumin are yet to begin.

There are weeks that fly by and this last week was one of them. I helped cater for the birthday lunch of a ninety-year-old. Ian had read a short story and a poem, and then reminded the guest of honour of all the things that had happened in the year in which she was born. She suddenly remembered so many things from her childhood and we all listened fascinated as she told of going to the dairy for milk, the Chinese garden where they bought their fresh vegetables, the ice cart that superseded the coolgardie safe. So many changes yet there she was, petite, vital, full of fun and a zest for living that would put to shame many younger than herself. That evening Ian was giving one of a series of three lectures on Tim Winton's *That Eye the Sky* and the following evening a lecture to a historical society. The following day we are to leave for the wedding, so I decide to stay at home and put out the suits, shirts, ties and so on for my husband and two grandsons and attend to all the last-minute things such as food for the sixteen-year-old who will be occupying the back seat.

The next morning it is cool and as we pack the flowers and our bucket into the car and put on the air conditioning I feel sure they will survive the journey. When we have settled into our motel I go to the church with my two brothers and their wives to see what vases will be available and to unwrap the flowers and give them some water and space to breathe before I arrange them the following morning. Our motel rooms overlook the lazy Edward River with its beautiful river gums and marvellous bird life. I feel as if I could just sit out on the balcony and do nothing for a week.

The church is modern, built only seventeen years ago with an enormous stained-glass window, soft sea-blue carpet and pine pews and flooded with light. Friends of the bride have offered their gardens for flowers and in the morning we will 'raid' the luxuriant gardens full of roses, day lilies and all the greenery we will need. These country women are so generous, so willing to cooperate in any way they can, such terrific gardeners.

By now it was seven-thirty and I realised I have not even had a cup of coffee. The restaurant we had intended to eat in had a muso's night in progress, with an audience of a hundred and twenty, so we repaired to the hotel that had been recommended. How these country people eat! We shared seafood platters that simply groaned with oysters, scallops, barramundi and prawns and a beautiful salad, served with fresh, warm bread and three different butters. Only Ian knew that this was something of a celebratory meal, for it was exactly twelve months ago to the day that I had my surgery. The meal was so reasonably priced and served by a young country girl with ease and charm. Because I have to be up early on my garden raids we settle for what is by now not an early night.

Ian and I wake with a very loud dawn chorus but soon go back to sleep until the alarm wakens us. The sky is cloudless and the air seems soft and dreamy like all Riverina mornings at this time of year. The bride's friend, Helen, and I collect an abundance of flowers and while the men fill the urns I and my sisters-in-law make identical arrangements with the flowers. I fill a vase with roses just under the altar where the area is floodlit and there are enough day lilies and golden roses to make a tall vase for the reception area. The bride is busy filling rose bowls for the tables and all seven of us get to work to set up tables and chairs ready for the caterers. There is just enough time to put our feet up for half an hour after our late lunch. I need that. My legs are aching after so much standing and walking.

The bride's father is recovering from a slight stroke but is determined to take his daughter down the aisle and formally hand her to the bridegroom. The bride looks beautiful in her elegant frock and an apple green fascinator in her hair. She carries cream roses and wears on a silver necklace the pearl I had given her. She and Peter only have eyes for each other and the clergyman is sensitive to both of them, leading them so gently through their vows. There are weddings and there are weddings at this point in the twenty-first century, but this is a traditional one. Peter's brother and a friend of the bride read from the Song of Solomon and an extract from *Captain Corelli's Mandolin* that seem to me to be just right for the occasion. David has the capacity to engage with an audience and he reads beautifully. I can't say it to anyone, of course, but I am so proud of these two handsome men, so very different in many ways, and so fond of each other. This is the first family wedding without my daughter and I have to stop my mind from thinking about it or I will never get through the day, but how I long to have Jane here, or even to know that she is well and happy. As the Buddhists say, it is the grit in the wheel. It all seems so crazy whenever I think about it, but the Widor toccata is booming out and the bridal couple walk together down the aisle followed by the bride's daughter and the bridegroom's son. The arts complex is by the side of a lake and they have decided to serve drinks and food on the lawns and go inside to what had been the old Anglican church for the speeches, toasts and cutting of the cake.

The moon is almost full. A perfect night for lovers and a reception. My legs give out before the evening is over and with some of the others I move inside to the comfort of a chair.

My son and daughter-in-law want a party for all the 'blood relations', as they put it, so the next day we are all in the garden under vines and shadecloth and being served a buffet lunch. I watch the newlyweds as they circulate from table to table, serve drinks and make everyone feel welcome. This is the first time many of them have met. People have come up from town and from properties some distance away so everyone is getting to know each other. But it all seems so relaxed and easy and I think what a wonderful host and hostess they are.

31

What have I discovered about myself and life in these last twelve months? Certainly I think I can separate the important from the unimportant. Just when I thought we could not possibly love each other any more I have found that Ian and I have never been closer. Our love making has an extra dimension to it because neither of us knows what the future will bring and we want to savour every minute of life. We don't entertain as much as we once did and there are times when I feel quite guilty about that, but to be together is enough. I read a poem of Elizabeth Bishop's entitled *One Art*. This was part of it:

> The art of losing isn't hard to master;
> so many things seem filled with the intent
> to be lost that their loss is no disaster.
>
> Lose something every day. Accept the fluster
> of lost door keys, the hour badly spent.
> The art of losing isn't hard to master.
>
> Then practice losing farther, losing faster:
> places, and names, and where it was you meant
> to travel. None of these will bring disaster.

I have read only recently that fighting cancer can be likened to guerilla warfare. 'The enemy lies hidden within your defences, difficult to detect and difficult to attack.' And it is certainly true that some days it does feel as if I am waging war against these unknowns, but one thing I have done in the past twelve months is to master the loss of my breast. I put on my bra with its prosthesis each morning and am conscious of the weight of it, but most days now that is the only time I think about my loss.

There was an item of news a few days ago about the restoration of the famous Frauenkirche in Dresden. When Ian and I were researching in Eastern Germany we had seen the enormous blocks of stone all numbered and lying in the area where the church would be rebuilt. We saw the church now in the news bulletin, extravagant in its gold and marble and marvelled at what could be made of seeming destruction. I am reminded of the adage, 'It isn't what happens to us in life. It is what we do with what happens to us.' That for me was, and still is, the challenge.

Epilogue
May 2006

It is eighteen months since my surgery and I have just heard an Encounter program on the ABC raising the question 'How happy can we be?' One of the participants in the discussion said that happiness is like a cat. If you try to coax or call it, it will never come. But if you pay no attention to it, you'll find it rubbing against your legs.

An Ethiopian says that the Ethiopian view of happiness is found in communal living and he finds it difficult to reconcile this with the western individualistic society where everyone talks about needing their own space. If, as I believe, the most important things in life are to be found in relationships, then I find myself agreeing with the Ethiopian.

In Ian McEwan's book *Saturday*, he has the surgeon reflect,

> It's a commonplace of parenting and modern genetics that parents have little or no influence on the characters of their children. You never know what you are going to get. Opportunities, health prospects, accent, table manners, these might lie within your power to shape, But who really determines the sort of person who's coming to live with you is which sperm finds which egg, how the cards in two packs are chosen, then how they are shuffled, halved and spliced at the moment of recombination.

He is musing on the difference between his eighteen-year-old son who is so unlike his sister, Daisy.

That is what family and community are all about, I think. That enormous diversity and the way we can be there for each other and grow ourselves as we try to understand them.

Age is not an issue for the Ethiopians. Even as I have been writing this I have been wondering whether my writing will be of any use to someone else in my situation. Our very uniqueness prevents us from being exactly like anyone else.

These last eighteen months have taken me on a strange journey. There are days when I give thanks for simply being alive, and can echo the words of the poet e.e.cummings:

> i thank You God for most this amazing
> day: for the leaping greenly spirits of trees
> and a blue true dream of sky; and for everything
> which is natural which is infinite which is yes

At other times I have to dig deep within myself to find a positive response to answer the challenges life brings. I want to make things better for my children and for my grandchildren, but I know that each of us has to climb our own mountain.

Time and the near future loom large for most people over their three score years and ten. At some time or other they ask, 'What did all this experience mean? What have I made of these experiences? What will I leave behind?' So often it all seems to have been so brief and at other times one crowded life filling and overflowing the glass. What strange creatures we are.

The Chinese say that nothing we do changes the past, but everything we do changes the future. I suppose I have been writing to offer something of my life and its experiences to other people rather as someone shows you small travel photos and you are able to say, 'Oh yes. I've been there.' Perhaps that is all we can do.

Just One Other Thing

It is now a little over two years since my breast cancer surgery. I am somewhat reluctant to write this final piece because I have tried to push from my mind any negative thoughts.

I haven't wanted to revisit my mastectomy. As I put on my bras each morning and take my Tamoxifen each evening, I have a constant reminder of my physical loss. But really these are little losses, little griefs.

Last Sunday was Transfiguration Sunday and our minister spoke of how in a Basil Fawlty fashion we often look for duck a l'orange in life when what we have is a messy flummery dish. She spoke too of how it is only when we dive into the deep parts of the ocean that we see its astonishing beauty. It came to me again how cancer surgery takes us to the depths.

A young friend said to me recently that I hadn't written very much about my religious faith in this account of my journey, and I felt rebuked, although this had not been her intention. I am aware of the great variety of religious experiences shared by people of all faiths and of the way in which their faith sustains them. I didn't want to claim that there is only one understanding of God. In my darkest moments my understanding of God as revealed in the life of Jesus is the God of my beginning and of my ending, the God who has been part of what I believe about life throughout all my experiences.

From early childhood, many of us can recite the 23rd Psalm but it is only when we 'walk through the valley of the shadow of death' that we are able to hold fast to what the theologian Paul Tillich described as 'the ground of our being'.

We all long for perfect endings in life, for everything to be tied up neatly, but the reality is that there are always so many loose ends. Faced with uncertainty we all share a great desire to tie those ends up. Every day I try to accept the things that I cannot change so that each day is enjoyed to the full.

There are always reasons for celebration. The twenty-first birthday of our eldest grandchild and the beginning of his university studies, the promotion of our eldest to a new position within the pastoral company where he is a manager, visits from our lovely granddaughter now living in Melbourne. I find that I am greedy for the love of my intimate family in a way I have never previously experienced. Sometimes I think they are rather bewildered by it all. Hasn't she always been able to manage? Why do little things upset her? Of course it requires a change of thinking on their part. I have passed my three score years and ten and for that I am grateful. But I won't be here for ever and perhaps they can learn from me that Buddhist idea of the impermanence of existence.

There are always signs of hope. Recently in an extract from *The Lancet* came the news of a new drug which, when taken alongside Tamoxifen two years after breast cancer may add seventeen per cent to the survival rate of patients. Lore Segal in an essay published in *Harper's Magazine* tells that when Pandora opened her box of calamities over the earth, there fell out a last straggler, hope. Hope is what sustains me in the night when flushed hot and unable to sleep my mind turns to the milestones, the transitions, the griefs of life.

That last straggler from Pandora's box I need. I know that I am not alone in this fight for survival. You only have to walk into a hospital to see the daily struggles of patients as they climb the hill to recovery.

Life involves mystery. We don't have answers to so many of the things that trouble us. But I am also often astounded by the sheer joy of being alive, of waking up to the sounds of magpies, feeling the warmth of the sun on my face and sharing all this with someone I have loved and who has loved me for over fifty years. This is such a passionate, affirming thing to experience. Cancer has enabled me to focus on the things that really matter, to separate the gold of life from the dross.

I wrote all this not knowing how much time on this earth is left to me, but with the hope that one day it may help someone get over *their* hurdle with courage, faith and hope.

Our dream of life will end as dreams do end, abruptly and completely, when the sun rises, when the light comes. All that fear and all that grief about nothing. But that cannot be true. I can't believe we will forget our sorrows altogether. That would mean forgetting we had lived, humanly speaking.

Sorrow seems to me to be a great part of the substance of human life…sometimes I almost forget my purpose in writing this, which is to tell you things I would have told you if you had grown up with me.

Marilynne Robinson, *Gilead*

www.ingramcontent.com/pod-product-compliance
Lightning Source LLC
Chambersburg PA
CBHW030909080526
44589CB00010B/213